Clinical Cases for MRCPCH Theory and Science

February 2014

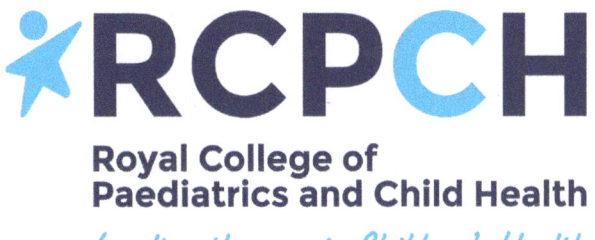

RCPCH

**Royal College of
Paediatrics and Child Health**

Leading the way in Children's Health

Foreword

We are delighted to see this new publication. In 2013 we launched the new examination focusing on Theory & Science. In the day of Evidence-based Medicine, the science, the research, the evidence that underpins our practice is vitally important. But how much should you know to pass our examination?

Will Carroll has brought together almost 40 different authors and created a very welcome learning resource. It does not set out to cover every detail of paediatric Theory & Science, but provides a wide spread of information from the baby to the child to the young person. Most helpfully, it gives our paediatric trainees some idea of the depth of knowledge which is expected.

No one can deny the importance of Theory & Science, everyone would agree it would have to be in our assessment strategy. We hope that you will find this a welcome aid to your learning if you are preparing for the Membership examination or if you simply wish to advance your knowledge of the science that we use in our everyday practice.

Congratulations and thank you to all who have contributed to this innovative new title.

Hilary Cass

President Royal College of Paediatrics and Child Health

Preface

I have been lucky enough to be involved with teaching throughout my career. I have also witnessed much teaching, good and bad. Whilst teaching was something I have always enjoyed, I never thought of it as a 'career'. However, 8 years ago, I was given the opportunity to take up a consultant role which combined teaching and paediatrics. I began to think more critically about what I had seen and done within teaching. I read and re-read the best textbooks I could find. I even read a little educational theory.

I came to the conclusion that the best teaching I had seen and done not only 'covered the basics' it related to more fundamental scientific principles. In a classroom of 20-30 students, some will always want only the bare minimum to get through the exams but most will be compelled by the physiology, pharmacology and anatomy of the topic. Congenital heart disease comes alive when the anatomy and embryology is understood and each student can follow the flow of blood through a normal and abnormal circulation. The host of syndromes seen in paediatrics are demystified by an understanding of the genetic principles which result in differing clinical phenotypes. Asthma and bronchiolitis are made exciting and memorable by an understanding of the lung physiology and anatomy. I also discovered how little was written about this science in typical textbooks and how quickly and often the science changes.

At the same time I became involved with the MRCPCH examinations team. Two years ago, small groups of us were asked to consider the place of each part of the MRCPCH written examination in training and subsequent practice. It became clear that MRCPCH Part 1B in particular lacked a clear focus or indeed syllabus to guide learners, this has now been rectified (1). After quite a bit of debate a new name and new syllabus was generated and so MRCPCH Part 1b underwent a metamorphosis into MRCPCH Theory and Science of Practice. At the same time we have removed a large portion of the existing question bank and set about the huge task of commissioning, writing and reviewing new and important questions.

The aim of this book is to illuminate how science can be used to tackle clinical cases in paediatrics. For the student who is unfamiliar with MRCPCH Theory and Science questions and the examination format this will exemplify the types of question asked in the actual exam. By reflecting the new syllabus it hopes to demonstrate to the reader how those who set the examination generate questions and then place them into the question bank and MRCPCH Theory and Science papers.

For those studying for the examination, we hope this short book will supplement your existing learning and that it will enable you to access some of the weightier textbooks and even the occasional scientific paper or recent review article. For those of you writing questions, I hope this will offer an insight into what makes a good question in the new format of the exam. For those like me, who enjoy understanding the science of what we see and teach I hope that this encourages you to think about what you see in clinical practice and relate this to your students of all ages and stages of their careers.

This small book is not intended to be read from cover to cover at one sitting. The 'fact heavy' nature of each chapter and the lack of illustrations in this first edition would make that very difficult. Rather, I would hope that readers will read a case, attempt the questions and then carefully read through the discussion that follows. This might prompt further reflection and sometimes further reading. Each chapter has been ruthlessly edited to ensure that it does not extend beyond 4 pages but do not underestimate the time you may need to successfully negotiate each chapter.

The very best questions in this book (and indeed in the exam) do not aim to test clinical experience, rather they are attempting to see if you understand why and how something happens. In short, have you developed your scientific knowledge sufficiently so that it can underpin your subsequent clinical practice?

I would like to offer heartfelt thanks to all the chapter authors for their enthusiasm patience and hard work. Most of all I want to thank my wife (also a contributor) and children for tolerating my negligence and fatigue during the preparation of this book.

Enjoy.

Dr Will Carroll

Chair of MRCPCH Written Exams   Derbyshire Children's Hospital September 2013

1. Appendices: Syllabus (Appendix 1). Found at: http://www.rcpch.ac.uk/sites/default/files/TheoryScience Practice_syll2013.pdf

Contents

Chapter 1: A girl with unequal pupils
Dr Will Carroll

A 7 old girl is admitted to the children's emergency department with acute severe asthma. She is treated with oral steroids, nebulised salbutamol and ipratropium bromide. After one hour she is not improving and you are called to review her. She is maintaining her airway, has a respiratory rate of 45 per minute with moderate intercostal and subcostal recessions. She has widespread wheeze with equal air entry bilaterally. Her trachea is central. Her heart rate is 150 per minute and her capillary refill time is 1 second. Her blood pressure is 110/65mmHg. She is sitting upright and responds to voice although she is tired and fretful. Her left pupil is 6mm and unreactive. Her right pupil is 3mm and reactive. Over the next hour she gradually improves clinically. As her respiratory distress settles, she wants to go to sleep but her pupils remain unequal. Her eye movements are normal, she can see through both eyes and fundoscopy is normal.

Q1. What is the most likely cause of unequal pupils?

A.   Horner's syndrome
B.   Ipratropium bromide
C.   Physiological anisocoria
D.   Salbutamol
E.   Undisclosed head injury

Q2. What should you do next?

A.   Administer cocaine eye drops
B.   Administer pilocarpine eye drops
C.   Arrange CT scan of the brain
D.   Reassure as this is physiological
E.   Undertake fluorescein-assisted examination of the cornea

Answers and Rationale

Q1. B. Ipratropium bromide
Q2. B. Administer pilocarpine eye drops

Like many clinical puzzles, the answer lies in an understanding of the science. To answer correctly we need to understand something of the anatomy of the eye and the physiology of pupillary size and reflexes. In this instance we also need to know the pharmacology of the drugs used to treat asthma. It is important to understand the determinants of pupillary size and the components of the pupillary reflexes as these are important in several uncommon but important conditions in childhood.

Pupillary size is determined by the contraction of the iris. The iris is a contractile structure consisting mainly of smooth muscle. Adult pupil size can change from 1-2 millimetres to 8 millimetres. This means that by changing the size of the pupil, the eye can change the amount of light that enters it by 30 times. The iris contains two groups of smooth muscles; a circular group called the sphincter pupillae which constrict the pupil and are under parasympathetic control, and radial group called the dilator pupillae which dilate the pupil and are under sympathetic control. The pupil will dilate in response to either sympathetic nerves from the superior cervical ganglion or by influx of circulating adrenaline.

The dilator pupillae is stimulated through α1-adrenoceptors. The relative β2-selective nature of salbutamol ensures that it has a negligible effect on pupillary size. Excess circulating catecholamines from respiratory distress may dilate the pupils but the effect would result in bilateral pupillary enlargement.

The sphincter pupillae is stimulated through M3-muscarinic acetylcholine receptors. M3-receptors are distributed widely, but are found particularly in the lungs and eye where they respectively provoke bronchospasm and pupillary constriction. Several commonly used medicines act as either agonists or antagonists on these receptors. Pilocarpine is a non-selective muscarinic receptor agonist which when administered as eye-drops acts therapeutically on the M3-muscarinic acetylcholine receptors within the eye. It has been used in the treatment of glaucoma for over 100 years. Pilocarpine causes contraction of both the iris and the ciliary muscle. Contraction of the ciliary muscle opens the trabecular meshwork which allows aqueous humour to leave the eye thus decreasing intraocular pressure. In our case, pilocarpine eye drops would have little or no effect on the abnormally dilated pupil (1). This is because ipratropium bromide has been blown into the left eye during nebulisation. Whilst I do not know how commonly this occurs in clinical practice, I have seen this twice myself in the last 5 years and it is widely reported in the literature (2-4). 0.32% of people reporting side-effects of using ipratropium bromide report unequal pupils. Ipratropium bromide (Atrovent) is a nonselective muscarinic antagonist (M1-5). Its principal therapeutic indication in childhood is in the treatment of acute severe asthma where it has proven benefits (5). It acts in the lungs on M3-muscarinic acetylcholine receptors opposing bronchoconstriction of smooth muscle and reducing mucus production of goblet cells. Ipratropium bromide does not diffuse into the blood thus limiting systemic side effects. This is in contrast to other non-selective muscarinic antagonists tolterodine, oxybutynin and atropine. These often also cause side effects of dry mouth, dry eyes, constipation, headache and sleepiness.

Physiological anisocoria is common and probably affects about 20% of the childhood population to some degree. It is more obvious in darker conditions and therefore is often detected when attempting fundoscopy. Whilst there are some exceptions, the vast majority of physiological anisocoria results in a difference in pupillary size of less than 1mm. Contraction anisocoria describes the tendency of the pupil of a directly illuminated eye to constrict more than the pupil of the contralateral eye. In 44 healthy children aged 6-16 years researchers found that illuminating the right eye led to larger contraction anisocoria than stimulating the left eye, and that right-side lateralization of contraction anisocoria was much greater in the boys than in the girls; the anisocoria produced was well less than 0.5 mm and not of clinical relevance (6). Red flags in children with anisocoria should include ptosis, anhidrosis (suggesting Horner's syndrome) and impaired eye movements. Our case has none of these.

Horner's syndrome results from a disruption of the sympathetic nervous supply to the eye at any point along its length. In Horner's syndrome, the pupil in the involved eye is usually smaller and does not dilate as well as the other eye. The child may have mild ptosis of the upper eyelid. A subtle but specific finding is the presence of an accompanying slight elevation of the lower eyelid (known as inverse ptosis). Because the upper eyelid is slightly lower than normal, and the lower eyelid is slightly higher than normal, the eye may appear smaller. If the Horner's syndrome developed during the first year of life, the iris on the affected side may appear lighter in colour than the uninvolved side. Sometimes, the pressure in the eye is lower in the Horner's eye and sometimes there is decreased sweating of the skin on the face on the affected side. The exogenous administration of cocaine eye drops can accurately distinguish between Horner's and physiological anisocoria in the majority of cases. Cocaine usually causes dilated pupils as it blocks reuptake of noradrenaline. Therefore a small pupil which does not dilate in response to cocaine eye drops has no sympathetic supply.

The pupillary reflex has afferent, central and efferent components. The afferent limb of the reflex is dependent upon retinal receptor cells, bipolar cells, ganglion cells and the optic nerve and tract. The central components are controlled by the pretectal nucleus in the midbrain and the Edinger-Westphal nucleus. Both the ipsilateral and contralateral Edinger-Westphal nuclei receive identical afferent input which causes the consensual light reflex. Parasympathetic stimulation of the sphincter pupillae is achieved via the oculomotor nerve. Distortion of the oculomotor nerve by raised intracranial pressure may result in initially an oval then non-reactive pupil on the ipsilateral side. This young girl can see through both eyes. Therefore defects in the afferent or central components of the reflex are highly unlikely. Her cooperation also makes a sudden undiagnosed intracranial injury unlikely and her normal eye movements almost certainly rule it out.

Corneal injury results in conjunctival injection and occasionally a reactive miosis. However, in the absence of other history and with such a large discrepancy in pupil size this is a highly unlikely cause for the signs described.

Syllabus Mapping

Ophthalmology

- know and understand the anatomy and embryology of the eye
- understand how the structure of the eye relates to function
- know the physiology of the eye and its movement, eg pupillary reflexes, anisocoria
- understand the pharmacology of agents commonly used in eye disease, including mydriatics

Respiratory medicine and ENT

- understand the pharmacology of agents commonly used in respiratory disease, eg asthma

References

1. Bond DW, Vyas H, Venning H. Mydriasis due to self-administered ipratropium bromide. *Eur J Pediatr* 2002;**161**:178.

2. Papalkar D, Sharma NS, Ooi JL, Sharma S, Francis IC. Pupil blown by a puffer. *Lancet* 2004; **364;** 415.

3   Weir REP, Whitehead DEJ, Zaidi FH, Greaves BBG. Pupil blown by a puffer. *Lancet* 2004;**363**:1853.

4. Iosson N. Nebulizer-associated anisocoria. *N Engl J Med* 2006;**354**:e8.

5. L Rodrigo GJ, Castro-Rodriguez JA. Anticholinergics in the treatment of children and adults with acute asthma: a systematic review with meta-analysis. *Thorax* 2005;**60** :740–746.

6. Fan X, Miles JH, Takahashi N, Yao G. Sex-specific lateralization of contraction anisocoria in transient pupillary light reflex. *Invest Ophthalmol Vis Sci.* Mar 2009;**50(3)**:1137-44.

Chapter 2: A little girl with persistent wheeze
Dr Arvind Shah, Dr Benita Morrissey

A 3 year old girl, Chloe, presents with recurrent episodes of viral induced wheeze. These began at the age of 2 years when she started at the local nursery. The episodes occur with upper respiratory tract infections; they last for up to five days and occur more frequently in the winter period. She was given salbutamol by her GP and responds well to this given via a spacer device. There is no response to antibiotics.

In between episodes, she is completely well with no cough, wheeze or difficulty breathing (interval symptoms) and she is growing normally. She has no allergies, and no history of eczema or allergic rhinitis. There is no family history of atopy. She is commenced on montelukast as preventative therapy.

Q1. Which one of these statements best describes the mechanism of action of montelukast?

A. Blocks the action of leukotriene D4 in the lung
B. Decreases the level of gamma interferon
C. Increases the level of leukotriene D4
D. Increases the level of phophodiesterase PDEIII
E. Inhibits C1 esterase enzymes

Q2. Which of the following is not a risk factor for the development of asthma at school age?

A. Allergic rhinitis
B. Breast-fed as infant
C. Food allergies
D. Obesity
E. Parental history of asthma

Answers and Rationale

Q1. A. Blocks the action of leukotriene D4 in the lung
Q2. B. Breast-fed as infant

By the age of six years nearly half of all children will have had at least one episode of wheeze (1). Most pre-school wheezing is associated with viral upper respiratory tract infections, which occur frequently in this age group. Asthma is less common and most with early wheeze will have stopped wheezing by school age. It is probably helpful to divide children with pre-school wheeze into one of two main phenotypes: Episodic (viral) wheeze and multi-trigger wheeze (2). Although viral wheeze is the commonest cause of wheezing in this age group a careful history and examination is needed to rule out other causes of wheezing in infants and young children (3).

Table 2.1: Causes, key clinical features and diagnostic investigations in childhood wheeze

Causes	Clinical features	Diagnostic investigations
Episodic viral wheeze or multi-trigger wheeze	Clear history of viral trigger (episodic) or multiple triggers	None needed if other causes excluded with history and examination
Viral infection/bronchiolitis	Coryza, bilateral crepitations and hyperinflation.	Nasopharyngeal aspirate for immunofluorescence/PCR
Gastro-oesophageal reflux disease /Recurrent aspiration	Vomiting, poor weight gain, recurrent chest infections	pH Study, bronchoscopy may show lipid laden macrophages, contrast study
Inhaled foreign body	Acute onset of symptoms with coughing or choking, sometimes focal wheeze	CXR, rigid bronchoscopy
Cystic Fibrosis	Cough in first few weeks of life, poor weight gain (if pancreatic insufficient)	Sweat test (may have been identified by newborn screening)
Primary ciliary dyskinesia	Rhinorrhea from young age, recurrent otitis media	CXR to look for dextrocardia (present in 50%,) ciliary studies
Immune Deficiency	Recurrent severe, persistent or unusual infections	Immunoglobulin's, B and T cells, functional antibodies, HIV test
Cardiac disease	Heart murmur, gallop rhythm, tachycardia, hepatomegaly, basal crepitations	CXR, ECG and echocardiogram
Post infectious bronchiolitis obliterans	History of previous viral infection (usually adenovirus)	High-resolution CT chest

Episodic viral wheeze is characterized by short episodes of wheeze associated exclusively with colds/ upper respiratory tract infections. Between episodes children are well and asymptomatic. The most common causative agents include rhinovirus, RSV (respiratory syncytial virus,) coronavirus, human metapneumovirus, parainfluenza and influenza. Episodes are more common in the winter. Episodic (viral) wheeze usually resolves by the age of six years, but it can continue or change into multiple-trigger wheeze. Multi-trigger wheeze resembles atopic asthma in older children with wheeze triggered not only by colds but also by non-viral triggers such as pets, running around and cold weather (2).

To overcome some of the limitations of a single 'point in time' description of wheezing episodes in childhood pre-school wheeze can also be described retrospectively as being transient (symptoms commence before three years and resolve by six years) persistent (symptoms continue beyond the age of six) and late-onset (symptoms that start after the age of three). Transient wheezers are thought to be born with airflow obstruction, whereas those with persistent wheeze (which may be episodic or multi-trigger, but more likely the latter) have normal lung function soon after birth, but lose lung function by age 4-6 years.

Airway obstruction in wheeze occurs as the result of small to moderate airway obstruction due to either inflammation or smooth muscle bronchoconstriction. A cellular inflammatory exudate with eosinophils, neutrophils, lymphocytes and mast cells can fill and obstruct the airways, and induce epithelial damage. Helper T lymphocytes and other immune cells produce proinflammatory cytokines such as IL4, IL5 and IL13. Thickening of the basement membrane has also been shown to occur, but is less prominent in pre-school wheeze than children with severe asthma. In episodic viral wheeze the bronchiolar lavage is mostly neutrophilic and blood studies done during wheezy episodes show neutrophilic rather than eosinophilic activation. This contrasts with atopic asthma in which the eosinophil dominates. It is therefore unsurprising that conventional asthma therapy is less likely to be helpful in this group. Treatment of episodic viral wheeze is aimed at parental education, reducing cigarette smoke exposure and use of short acting β-2 agonists when required. β-2 receptors are present and functional from infancy within the bronchioles. They act through activation of adenylyl cyclase and this increases intracellular cyclic AMP leading to relaxation of constricted bronchial smooth muscle. It has no effect on inflammation.

No treatment has been found to be disease modifying in episodic wheeze (1-5). However if children are having frequent or particularly severe episodes of viral wheeze preventative therapy should be considered. Montelukast has been shown in some studies to reduce the frequency of exacerbations by 30% and improve symptoms. Montelukast is a cysteinyl leukotriene receptor antagonist, and blocks the action of leukotriene D4 in the lungs and bronchial airways. The cysteinyl leukotrienes (leukotriene C4 D4 and E4) are important mediators of wheeze causing bronchoconstriction, vascular permeability and mucus secretion due to the release of inflammatory mediators from alveolar macrophages, eosinophils and mast cells. Montelukast blocks these actions and also has been reported to have some secondary anti-inflammatory properties reducing neutrophilic activation.

Regular maintenance dose inhaled corticosteroids have not been shown to reduce hospital admissions or oral corticosteroid courses in children with episodic viral wheeze, but a three month trial may be considered in some children who do not respond to Montelukast. They act by binding to glucocorticoid receptors and reducing airway inflammation. Multi-trigger wheeze in pre-school children should be treated as atopic asthma in older children, with a trial of inhaled corticosteroids.

In most children with episodic viral wheeze, symptoms will have resolved by school age. Risk factors for asthma in childhood include parental asthma, personal history of atopy (eczema, allergic rhinitis, food allergies) male sex, cigarette smoke exposure, low birth weight, obesity and airway hyper reactivity.

Being breast fed as a baby reduces this risk.

Syllabus Mapping

Infection, immunity & Allergy

*   know the epidemiology and natural history of atopic disease.

Respiratory Medicine

*   understand the physiological, pathophysiological and histological changes that occur in respiratory disease
*   know the genetic and environmental factors in the aetiology of respiratory diseases and disorders of the ears, nose and throat
*   understand the pharmacology of agents commonly used in respiratory disease

References and Further Reading

1.   Bhatt J, Smyth AR. A clinical approach to a wheezy infant. *Paediatr and Child Health 2012;* **22**:307-309.

2.   Brand PL, et al. Definition, assessment and treatment of wheezing disorders in preschool children: an evidence-based approach. *Eur Respir J* 2008;**32**:1096–1110.

3.   Bush A. The problem of preschool wheeze: new developments, new questions. *Acta Medica Lituanica* 2010;**17**:40-50.

4.   Grigg J. Wheeze in a pre-school child. *Paediatr and Child Health 2009;***20**:186-187.

5.   Liu A, Covar R *et al.* Chapter 38: Childhood Asthma. In; Kliegman RM, Stanton BMD, Geme J et al. Nelson Textbook of Pediatrics. 19th ed. Philadelphia, Elsevier Saunders; 2011.

Chapter 3: A child with poorly controlled asthma
Dr Rossa Brugha, Dr Will Carroll

An 8 year old Caucasian girl has been treated for asthma for the past three years by her GP with inhaled salbutamol and an inhaled corticosteroid (beclometasone dipropionate 200 mcg BD). Despite this she has recently had a worsening of her symptoms, and has been referred for a paediatric opinion. She is otherwise healthy apart from mild flexural eczema. There is no history of prematurity or significant respiratory infections. Her spirometry is:

	FEV_1(L)	%predicted	z-score	FVC (L)	%predicted	z-score
Pre bronchodilator	1.35	87.3	-0.96	1.65	95.6	-0.34
15 minutes post bronchodilator	1.52	98.3	-0.13	1.66	96.2	-0.29

Q1. Which physiological process best explains the observed bronchodilator response?

The bronchodilator response leads to:

A.   A reduction in gas viscosity

B.   Contraction of airway smooth muscle, which increases the velocity of exhaled gases

C.   Decreased goblet cell hyperplasia and mucus production

D.   Increased effort, resulting in a greater FEV_1 as a "learning effect" when performing spirometry

E.   Relaxation of airway smooth muscle increasing airway calibre

Further history reveals that her asthma symptoms worsen when she has coughs and colds. Her mother is very concerned about side effects, particularly about possible growth suppression with steroids. You decide to adjust her treatment medication and you want to outline the possible side effects to her and her mother.

Q2. Which is an appropriate medication choice, coupled with the correct side effect, from the treatment options outlined below?

A.   Alternate day oral prednisolone. Side effect – iatrogenic Cushing's disease

B.   Combination long acting bronchodilator and inhaled steroid (e.g. Seretide). Side effect – increased growth velocity

C.   Leukotriene receptor antagonist (e.g. Montelukast). Side effect – sleep disturbance or nightmares

D.   Slow release theophylline (e.g. Slo-phyllin). Side effect – bradycardia

E.   Stop her inhaled corticosteroid and start a long-acting inhaled bronchodilator (e.g. Salmeterol). Side effect – increased risk of sudden death

Answers and Rationale

Q1. E. Relaxation of airway smooth muscle increasing airway calibre
Q2. C. Leukotriene receptor antagonist (e.g. Montelukast). Side effect – sleep disturbance or nightmares

The first part of the question tests a candidate's knowledge of the pharmacology of salbutamol. Assessing the bronchodilator response (BDR) is one method of determining whether airway smooth muscle is contracted at rest. A positive response suggests that there is airway hyperresponsiveness which could be confirmed using either a metacholine challenge, exercise test or cold air challenge. The British Thoracic Society asthma guidelines advise that "bronchodilator responsiveness, peak expiratory flow variability or tests of bronchial hyper-reactivity may be used to confirm the diagnosis, with the same reservations as in adults". In this scenario there is bronchodilator responsiveness of 11%. 9% is reported as an appropriate cut-off point for a positive test in children (1).

The question requires the candidate to have prior knowledge that salbutamol is used to elicit bronchodilation in the test. While most candidates should be aware of this, it is possible to answer the question without prior knowledge as the question refers to a 'bronchodilator' and a candidate should know that bronchodilators predominantly act on bronchial smooth muscle to increase airway diameter. Airway resistance for laminar flow is described by Poiseuille's equation:

$$\text{Resistance} = \frac{8 \times \text{length} \times \text{viscosity of the gas}}{\pi \times (\text{radius})^4}$$

It predicts that airway resistance increases most dramatically as diameter decreases. However, most resistance to airflow is offered by the trachea and larger bronchi. This counterintuitive observation is due to the branching of the trachea-bronchial tree which ensures the combined cross-sectional area of the smallest airways is sufficiently large to provide very little resistance to flow. At the 23rd airway generation, which are 0.4 mm in diameter the total cross-sectional area is 4 m^2 because there are 300 million airways of this size. In contrast the tracheal cross-sectional area is just 3 cm^2. Corticosteroids do reduce mucus production but not in the short period of time outlined – and would not account for the improvement in FEV_1 in just 15 minutes.

The first 25-35% of expiration which includes the PEFR is effort dependent. By contrast the remaining two-thirds or the flow volume curve is largely effort independent. Once a child makes >90% effort then the values for FEV_1 and FEF_{25-75} are predominantly flow-dependent rather than effort dependent. Whilst there is often improvement seen between first and second attempts, attempts are only considered valid if three attempts within 10% of each other are achieved. Once a consistent score is achieved by a cooperative child then you can be sure that a child is making a good effort. The FVC in the test scenario is unchanged, a further indicator of similar efforts in both pre- and post bronchodilator attempts.

Although gas viscosity does influence airway resistance, salbutamol does not significantly alter gas viscosity. Increased air flows can be achieved by using a mixture of helium and oxygen. Heliox (helium oxygen mixtures) can be useful in severe upper airway obstruction.

The second part of the question aims to test a candidate's knowledge of the possible side effects of asthma medications. Following their introduction, long acting beta agonists (LABAs) were associated with sudden death in children over 12 and adults with asthma (3) but this was only in the context of using a LABA without inhaled steroid (4). Despite mother's concerns it would be inappropriate to stop her inhaled steroids. This child has poorly controlled (symptomatic) asthma and a significant bronchodilator response (which confirms the diagnosis of asthma). Therefore careful reassurance about the known effects of low dose inhaled corticosteroids are required. Versus placebo, inhaled budesonide results in a 1.2cm loss in adult height (5). If a LABA is used then it is important to ensure that inhaled corticosteroids are continued. One way to ensure this is to use a combination inhaler.

All of the other options would be likely to improve asthma control, however the paired side effects for stem B and D are incorrect. Inhaled steroids decrease growth velocity (6), and phosphodiesterase inhibitors such as theophylline cause tachycardia, not bradycardia.

Thus the candidate only really has a choice between using a leukotriene receptor antagonist or alternate day oral steroids. High leukotriene levels have been found in patients with asthma. Cysteinyl leukotrienes (C4, D4 and E4) are derived from arachidonic acid with the help of the enzyme 5 lipoxygenase; this inflammatory pathway is not modified by corticosteroids hence the scientific basis for the use of LTRAs. Cysteinyl leukotrienes increase mucus production, bronchoconstriction, eosinophil recruitment and exudation of plasma –all being inflammatory processes. Cysteinyl LTRAs (montelukast is the only one licensed for use in children) have been shown to modify the above processes. The advantage of montelukast is that it is a once-daily medication either in granule form for use in the 6-24 month age range or as a pink chewy cherry-flavoured tablet in children over 2 years. It is effective in allergic asthma and in viral-induced wheeze in some young children. Whilst this is a valuable treatment and frequently well tolerated and easy to administer it is important to be aware of the two common side effects, sleep disturbance and increased thirst. Upon initiation parents must be informed about possible side effects (7).

Corticosteroids pass through the cell membrane of many inflammatory cells and the structural cells within the lung, probably by diffusion. In the cytoplasm they attach themselves to glucocorticoid receptors and form complexes which then translocate into the cell nucleus. Here they bind to specific genes involved with inflammation resulting in increased transcription of genes which suppress and reduce transcription of those which enhance airway inflammation. By non-genomic processes they may also inhibit inflammatory factors such as Nuclear Factor kappa B (NFκB) and Activator Protein 1. Corticosteroids are clinically very helpful as they reverse airway hyper-reactivity, a process which takes place within epithelial cells and which, if not treated early, leads to chronic inflammation and subsequent permanent remodelling of the airways, a process which is non-reversible and produces fixed airways changes.

Whilst alternate day oral steroids are highly likely to be effective, side effects are also very likely particularly when used for more than a few days. These include weight gain, muscle weakness, abnormal fat deposition, striae, acne, osteoporosis, hypertension, glaucoma, cataracts and significant reduction in growth velocity in childhood. Further details about the physiological consequence of long term oral steroids can be found in Chapter 14.

Syllabus Mapping

Respiratory medicine and ENT

* be able to interpret and select appropriate respiratory investigations, e.g. blood gases, spirometry, body plethysmography, transfer factor
* understand the pharmacology of agents commonly used in respiratory disease, e.g. asthma, infections

References and Further Reading

1. Dundas, I, et al. Diagnostic accuracy of bronchodilator responsiveness in wheezy children. *Thorax* 2005;**60**(1):13-16.

2. Levy, ML, et al. Summary of the 2008 BTS/SIGN British guideline on the management of asthma. *Prim Care Respir J*, 2009;**18 Suppl** 1:S1-16.

3. Nelson, HS. *et al.* The Salmeterol Multicenter Asthma Research Trial: a comparison of usual pharmacotherapy for asthma or usual pharmacotherapy plus salmeterol. *Chest 2006*;**129**(1):15-26.

4. Sears, MR. The FDA-mandated trial of safety of long-acting beta-agonists in asthma: finality or futility? *Thorax* 2012;**2**:2.

5. Kelly, HW. *et al.* Effect of inhaled glucocorticoids in childhood on adult height. *N Engl J Med* 2012;**367(10)**:904-12.

6. Martinez, FD. et al. Use of beclomethasone dipropionate as rescue treatment for children with mild persistent asthma (TREXA): a randomised, double-blind, placebo-controlled trial. *Lancet* 2011;**377(9766)**:650-7.

7. Wallerstedt, SM. et al. Montelukast and psychiatric disorders in children. *Pharmacoepidemiol Drug Saf* 2009;**18(9)**:858-64.

Chapter 4: The catarrhal child
Dr Amelia Saunders, Dr Will Carroll

An 11 year old boy presents to your clinic having recently moved to the region from elsewhere in the UK. He has a long history of troublesome cough. He developed respiratory distress shortly after birth following a pregnancy complicated by maternal Group B Strep carriage. He was treated with antibiotics and required oxygen for 2 weeks. Over the first 6 months of life he was 'in and out' of hospital with further respiratory illnesses, each time requiring oxygen. Throughout life he has persistent rhinitis a blocked nose and a wet sounding cough. He had glue ear but mum declined grommet insertion and instead elected for hearing aids, which he wore until 5 years of age. At this time a diagnosis of asthma was made on clinical grounds. He is currently treated with a long-acting beta agonist/inhaled steroid combined inhaler and leukotriene receptor antagonist but remains symptomatic. Examination reveals a well-grown boy with a wet sounding, low-pitched cough with normal heart sounds and no murmurs.

Q1. Which part of the respiratory tract is most likely to be abnormal?

A.   Alveoli
B.   Bronchial smooth muscle
C.   Cilia
D.   Goblet cells
E.   Vocal cords

Q2. What is the most appropriate investigation to screen for the suspected condition?

A.   Chest X-ray
B.   Nasal exhaled nitric oxide
C.   Pulmonary function tests
D.   Saccharin test
E.   Sweat testing

Answers and Rationale

Q1. C. Cilia
Q2. B. Nasal exhaled nitric oxide

By understanding the basic function of human cilia, the clinical signs and symptoms of Primary Ciliary Dyskinesia (PCD) can be easily understood. The human respiratory tract is lined by epithelial cilia (1). Depending on the position within the human body cilia maybe motile or non-motile. Motile cilia are found in the upper and lower respiratory tract, in the reproductive tracts and ependymal lining of the brain (1,2).

A layer of mucus lines the respiratory tract, where inhaled particles become trapped. This forms one of the many defense mechanisms of the lung. Each ciliated epithelial cell has around 200 surface cilia, required for effective mucociliary clearance. To move mucus proximally to the oropharynx, cilia must be adequate in number, beat in coordination, beat to the correct frequency (5-20 Hz), and have an appropriate waveform (1). In PCD the primary defect may be in the function or structure of cilia, resulting in absent or abnormal motility, the consequence of such is mucus retention throughout the respiratory tract that subsequently tends to becomes infected (3). Table 4.1 shows clinical features of PCD (4).

Table 4.1: Clinical manifestations of PCD at different ages during childhood

Age	Clinical Manifestation
Neonatal period	• Signs of Respiratory Distress shortly after birth (hypoxia, tachypnoea, grunting, cough) • Rarely respiratory failure • Sinus inversus totalis (in 50% of cases – see below) • Rhinorrhoea/nasal congestion from day 1 of life • Hydrocephalus (dysfunctional edendymal cilia)
Infants and young children	• Chronic Sinusitis • Persistent nasal discharge • Chronic serous otitis media or persistent otorrhoea after insertion of tympanostomy tube (grommets) • Conductive hearing loss • Recurrent otitis media with effusion • Chronic moist cough (atypical asthma) • Recurrent pneumonia • Bronchiectasis • Nasal polyps and halitosis
Older children / Adolescents	• Same as for infants and young children • Chronic mucopurlent sputum production • Obstructive/mixed pattern on pulmonary function tests • Bronchiectasis more apparent in adolescence • Male infertility • Female infertility or ectopic pregnancy

In patients with PCD mutations in ciliary proteins are frequently found (2,3).

Cilia have a complex structure and are composed of more than 200 proteins, where 9 microtubular doublets are arranged in a ring, surrounding 2 central microtubules. Accessory proteins and intertubular connections maintain the cilial ultrastructure.

PCD has an incidence of between 1 in 15,000-30,000 live births and is mainly inherited as an autosomal recessive condition. Cilial function is vital for normal respiratory tract function. Symptoms of PCD are often present from birth, demonstrating that cilia have an important role in clearing fluid during the first few hours of life (1). The signs of respiratory distress following delivery will frequently be attributed to more common causes such as transient tachypnoea of the newborn or sepsis. Normal cilial function is required to determine laterality of the heart and abdominal organs, without it laterality occurs randomly, hence 50% of PCD patients exhibit sinus inversus totalis (2). In these children diagnosis often occurs at a much younger age. Any patient with sinus inversus totalis seen on X-ray should have further investigations to exclude PCD (4).

Diagnosis of PCD in children without dextrocardia is frequently delayed, as the symptoms seen in the first few years of life are often seen in young children. Commonly employed investigations may not immediately point to a diagnosis of PCD. Chest X-ray appearances range from completely normal to showing bronchiectasis or atelectasis (1). Pulmonary function tests maybe normal during early years, but as frequent infections ensue, an obstructive pattern maybe seen in later years. Often lung function remains stable, but in a proportion of patients function will continue to decline (3).

In healthy subjects high levels of nitric oxide (NO) are produced in the human nose and paranasal sinuses (5). Levels of exhaled nasal NO can be easily measured by non-invasive techniques. Exhaled nasal NO levels have been found to be uniformly very low in PCD patients and this can be clinically useful when diagnosing the disease. As a clinical investigation for PCD, exhaled nasal nitric oxide (NO) has very high sensitivity and specificity, making it an attractive screening test, prior to confirmatory testing in children over 5 years of age (5). This has supplanted the saccharin test which measures the time taken for a pellet of saccharin placed on the inferior turbinate to be tasted (normal= <30 minutes) (6). Limitations of the saccharin test includes poor sensitivity and specificity and it is therefore not recommended as a screening test for PCD.

For completeness, sweat testing should be performed and immunoglobulin levels measured. This aims to exclude respiratory conditions, such as cystic fibrosis and immunodeficiencies (3). Patients should be referred to specialist centers for definitive testing, to confirm PCD. To analyze the structure and function a nasal brushing or bronchoscopy can be used to obtain a sample of respiratory ciliated epithelia (4). The ciliary beat pattern and frequency is analsyed using video recording and electron microscopy. Whilst genetics behind PCD are currently being unraveled, genetic analysis is not recommended for initial diagnosis (1, 4).

The main aim of treatment is to maintain lung function and prevent further decline. Treatment for respiratory infection is similar to that advocated for cystic fibrosis. As defects in cilia cannot be corrected airway clearance techniques, such as chest physiotherapy, are used to aid mucus clearance.(4).

Syllabus Mapping

Respiratory Medicine and ENT

*   understand the physiological, pathophysiological and histological changes that occur in respiratory disease
*   be able to interpret and select appropriate respiratory investigations
*   understand the scientific basis of non-pharmacological interventions in respiratory disease, eg physiotherapy

References

1. Stillwell PC, Wartchow EP, Sagel SD. Primary Ciliary Dyskinesia in Children: A Review for Pediatricians, Allergists, and Pediatric Pulmonologists. *Pediatr Allergy Immunol Pulmonol* 2011;**24(4):**191-196.

2. Afzelius BA. *Cilia-related diseases.* J Pathol **2004;204:470–477.**

3. Hughes, D. Primary Ciliary Dyskinesia. *Paediatr Child Health* 2008;**13(8)**:672-674.

4. Barbato A, Frischer T, Kuehni CE, Snijders D, Azevedo I, Baktai G, et al. Primary ciliary dyskinesia: a consensus statement on diagnostic and treatment approaches in children. *Eur Respir J 2009;***34(6)***:1264-76.*

5. Read A. et al. An Official ATS Clinical Practice Guideline: Interpretation of Exhaled Nitric Oxide Levels (FE$_{NO}$) for Clinical Applications. *Am J Respir Crit Care Med* 2011;**184**:602-615.

6. Bush A, O'Callaghan C. Primary Ciliary Dyskinesia. *Arch Dis Child* 2002;**87**:363-365.

Chapter 5: The blue newborn
Dr Benita Morrisey, Dr Arvind Shah

You are called to see a baby who is 1 hour old. She was born by vaginal delivery at 38 weeks gestation, after an uncomplicated pregnancy. Mother has a history of depression, and was on fluoxetine throughout pregnancy. She was born in good condition and there were no risk factors for sepsis. The midwife is concerned that the baby looks blue. You check the baby's oxygen saturations and discover they are 65% in the left foot.

Q1. Which is the best descriptor of fetal circulation in the newborn?

A.   Blood flows through the foramen ovale from left atrium to right atrium
B.   In the fetus there are two umbilical arteries and one umbilical vein
C.   Over 90% of blood bypasses the liver via the ductus venosus
D.   The umbilical artery carries oxygenated blood from the placenta to the fetus
E.   The patency of the ductus arteriosus is maintained by the vasodilating effects of prostaglandin G2

Q2. Which stimuli would cause the pulmonary arterioles to constrict and lead to an increase in pulmonary vascular resistance?

A.   Capillary refill time of 2 seconds
B.   High blood oxygen levels (high pO_2)
C.   High blood pH
D.   Hypothermia
E.   Low blood carbon dioxide level (low pCO_2)

Q3. Which of the following is correct about fetal haemoglobin (HbF)?

A.   2,3 DPG levels are high in HbF as compared to adult haemoglobin
B.   Acidosis shifts the oxygen dissociation curve to the right
C.   The affinity of adult haemoglobin towards oxygen is greater than that of HbF
D.   The oxyhaemoglobin dissociation curve for HbF is shifted to the left as compared with adult haemoglobin
E.   The shift from HbF to HbA happens during adolescence

Answers and Rationale

Q1. **B. In the fetus there are two umbilical arteries and one umbilical vein**

Q2. **D. Hypothermia**

Q3. **D. The oxyhaemoglobin dissociation curve for HbF is shifted to the left as compared with adult haemoglobin.**

The normal fetal circulation

Oxygenated blood from the placenta returns to the fetus through the single umbilical vein. Approximately half will travel through the liver with an almost equal amount bypassing the liver, via the ductus venosus, into the inferior vena cava (IVC). The IVC also drains blood returning from the lower trunk and extremities.

In the right atrium blood from the upper body from the superior vena cava, with lower oxygen saturation, passes through the tricuspid valve into the right ventricle and the pulmonary artery. In-utero there is high pulmonary vascular resistance, and low systemic vascular resistance.

Consequently most blood travelling into the pulmonary artery (PA) is shunted across the ductus arteriosus (DA) into the descending aorta. The ductus arteriosus is a similar diameter to the descending aorta. Its patency is maintained by the low oxygen tension in the blood and the dilating effect of prostaglandin E2 produced by the placenta. This relatively deoxygenated blood then travels back to the placenta via the two umbilical arteries, which arise from the internal iliac arteries, to re-oxygenate. The relatively oxygenated blood from the IVC preferentially crosses the foramen ovale (FA) allowing blood to pass from the right atrium into the left atrium and left ventricle to supply the upper body, including the brain. Because of this pattern of flow in the right atrium the highly oxygenated blood preferentially supplies the brain, and the deoxygenated blood is shunted back to the placenta.

Fetal haemoglobin and the oxygen dissociation curve

In the fetus haemoglobin is in the form of fetal haemoglobin (HbF) which is made up of two alpha chains and two gamma chains. During the third trimester, the fetus starts to produce adult Hb (HbA – two alpha chains and two beta chains). By birth, the baby has around 80% HbF and 20% HbA. The gamma chains of HbF have reduced binding to 2,3 diphosphoglycerate (2,3 DPG). The reduced levels of 2,3 DPG in HbF causes the oxyhaemoglobin dissociation curve to be shifted to the left. This means that for a given pO_2 a higher proportion of HbF will be saturated with oxygen than HbA. The higher affinity of HbF for oxygen makes it easier for them to acquire oxygen from the maternal circulation. Alkalosis, hypocarbia (low pCO_2) and hypothermia also shift the oxygen dissociation curve to the left. After birth levels of 2,3 DPG rise rapidly, shifting the oxygen dissociation curve to the right, and helping red blood cells to unload oxygen more effectively to the tissues, and meet the increased metabolic requirements.

Changes at Birth and the Transitional Circulation

At birth when an infant takes its first breath, the lungs expand and the pulmonary vascular resistance falls rapidly. As a result blood starts to flow into the lungs and the increased pulmonary blood flow back to the left atrium causes functional closure of the foramen ovale. Occlusion of the umbilical cord removes the low resistance capillary bed and results in an increase in the systemic vascular resistance. Functional closure of the ductus arteriosus usually occurs within the first twenty-four to forty-eight hours after birth and is facilitated by the loss of prostaglandins from the placenta, reduced sensitivity of the ductus to prostaglandins and an increased pO2 after the onset of breathing. Anatomical closure of the ductus arteriosus usually occurs within 3 weeks.

Prior to birth the pulmonary blood vessels have a thick layer of smooth muscle, which plays a key role in pulmonary vasoconstricton. After birth, this muscle begins to thin and becomes less sensitive to changes in oxygenation. Any clinical situation that causes hypoxia, especially in the first few hours of life, with pulmonary vasoconstriction and a subsequent increase in pulmonary vascular resistance, can cause a delay in these normal circulatory changes potentiating right-to-left shunting across the ductus arteriosus and foramen ovale. This is known as persistent pulmonary hypertension of the newborn.

Cyanosis in the Newborn and Persistent pulmonary hypertension of the Newborn

Cyanosis occurs when arterial blood contains more than 5g/dL of deoxygenated haemoglobin. Cyanosis in newborn babies can be caused by a number of pathologies including respiratory causes; cardiac causes (cyanotic congenital cardiac disease,) persistent pulmonary hypertension of the newborn and other rarer causes such as methaemoglobinaemia.

Respiratory causes include severe respiratory distress syndrome (RDS) meconium aspiration syndrome, pneumonia, pneumothorax, and congenital lung problems such as pulmonary hypoplasia and congenital diaphragmatic hernia. Congenital cardiac disease occurs in 5-8/1000 live births. Cardiac causes of cyanosis usually present in the first few days of life and include transposition of the great arteries, tetralogy of Fallot with pulmonary atresia, pulmonary atresia, tricuspid atresia, Ebstein's anomaly, truncus arteriosus and total anomalous pulmonary venous drainage.

Persistent pulmonary hypertension of the newborn occurs predominantly in term and post-term babies. Predisposing factors include perinatal asphyxia, meconium aspiration syndrome, respiratory distress syndrome, early onset neonatal sepsis, polycythemia, hypoglycemia, hypothermia, maternal use of non-steroidal inflammatory drugs, maternal use of selective serotonin reuptake inhibitors, (such as fluoxetine) in the third trimester, and pulmonary hypoplasia due to diaphragmatic hernia or oligohydramnios.

Hypoxia, hypothermia, acidosis and hypoglycemia all trigger constriction of the pulmonary vasculature and a consequent increase in pulmonary vascular resistance. Often a vicious cycle ensues as increased pulmonary resistance and shunting reduces blood flow to the lungs and oxygenation resulting in worsening hypoxia and pulmonary vasoconstriction. Commonly babies with persistent pulmonary hypertension are very unwell and require full neonatal intensive care: ventilation to improve oxygenation, inotropic support to improve blood pressure and perfusion and pulmonary vasodilators such as nitric oxide. Many will go on to require other ventilator support such as high frequency oscillation ventilation, and some will require extracorporeal membrane oxygenation (ECMO).

Syllabus Mapping

Cardiology

•   know the normal fetal circulation and transitional changes after birth
•   understand the pathophysiology of cardiac conditions, including cyanosis

Neonatology

•   understand the normal physiological processes occurring during the perinatal period
•   understand the scientific basis of common diseases and conditions affecting the newborn

References

1.   Berhrsin J, Gibson A. Cardiovascular system adaptation at birth. *Paediatr and Child Health* 2010;**21(1)**:1-6.

2.   Carlo WA, Chapter 95 – Respiratory Tract Disorders In; Kliegman RM, Stanton BMD, Geme J et al. Nelson Textbook of Pediatrics. 19th ed. Philadelphia, Elsevier Saunders; 2011.

3.   Rudolph AM, Congenital cardiovascular malformations and the fetal circulation. *Arch Dis Child* 2010;**95:2**:F132-F136.

Chapter 6: Another blue child
Dr Rana Alia, Dr Talal Ezzo

A 9 year old boy who has recently arrived in the UK is referred by his GP for evaluation of a heart murmur. He complains of shortness of breath and blue lips on moderate exertion. On examination he plots between the 2nd and 9th centile for height and weight. He has no dysmorphic features. His heart rate is 110 beats per minute, blood pressure is 115/70 mmHg and oxygen saturations in air are 90%. He has a right ventricular heave, laterally displaced apex, loud second heart sound in the left upper sternal edge, a 2/6 pan-systolic murmur in the left sternal edge which is heard throughout the chest.

Q1.   Which ONE answer best describes the most likely cause of the heart murmur?

A.   Atrial septal defect
B.   Fallot's tetralogy
C.   Large ventricular septal defect
D.   Patent ductus arteriosus
E.   Small ventricular septal defect

Q2.   Concerning the second heart sound which of the following statements are true (T) or false (F)?

A.   It is generated by closure of the atrioventricular valves
B.   It is quieter in children with pulmonary hypertension
C.   The splitting decreases in children with ventricular septal defects
D.   The splitting increases in children with atrial septal defects
E.   The splitting is decreased by inspiration

Q3.   Which of the following statements concerning the ECG are true (T) or false (F)?

A.   The electrical impulse starts in the sinoatrial node in the wall of the left atrium
B.   The PR interval is the time between the onset of atrial depolaraistaion and the onset of ventricular depolarisation
C.   The T wave represents the period between the end of ventricular repolarisation and the beginning of atrial depolarisation
D.   Ventricular repolarisation is represented by the QRS complex
E.   Ventricular depolarisation produces T wave

Q4.   Which ONE of the following statements is most likely to be correct regarding the ECG findings in this patient?

A.   A dominant R wave in lead V1 is an indication of right ventricular hypertrophy
B.   A mean frontal QRS axis of >90° indicates left axis deviation
C.   It will be normal
D.   Q waves will be present in anterior chest leads (V1-V4)
E.   The P waves will be shortened and narrow

Answers and Rationale

Q1. C. Large ventricular septal defect
Q2. A. False. B. False. C. False. D. True. E. False
Q3. A. False. B. True. C. False. D. False. E. False
Q4. A. A dominant R wave in lead V1 is an indication of right ventricular hypertrophy

The first question in this case is quite clinical but maps well to the syllabus for the MRCPCH Theory and Science exam. It sets the scene nicely for more testing questions concerning a child with pulmonary hypertension and a large ventricular septal defect (VSD).

VSD is the most common form of congenital heart disease (25%). VSD initially causes a left to right shunt and the size of the shunt depends on the size of the VSD and the level of the pulmonary resistance compared to the systemic resistance. In large VSD (nonrestrictive), the pressure is equal in the right and left ventricles and the ratio of the pulmonary to systemic resistance determines the shunt size and direction. After birth, the pulmonary resistance falls and the size of the left to right shunt increases causing symptoms of heart failure. When the pulmonary pressure increases to equalize the systemic pressure, the shunt will become bidirectional and Eisenmenger syndrome can develop. In small VSDs (pressure restrictive), the right ventricle pressure is normal and the size of the defect limits the size of the shunt.

Large left to right shunt reduces the effective cardiac output, and the body compensates by increasing its intravascular volume and end diastolic volume. This volume overload can cause pulmonary congestion and symptoms of heart failure. The VSD murmur is usually loud and harsh in small defects due to the significant pressure gradient across the defect, while in large defects, there is no pressure gradient and the murmur will be quieter.

The ECG is usually normal in small VSD or it may show signs of left ventricular hypertrophy. In a large VSD, the ECG shows left and right ventricular hypertrophy and if there is pulmonary hypertension, the P wave will be tall. In larger VSDs the CXR may show signs of pulmonary congestion and cardiomegaly. Echocardiography is important to confirm the diagnosis and it will show the position and size of the defect. It can be used to estimate the shunt size and the pulmonary pressure, and to exclude any other abnormalities. The cardiac catheter is not important for the diagnosis and should be considered only if added information is needed or to assess the pulmonary resistance.

Examination in the assessment of the cardiovascular system

Cardiac auscultation forms one part of the cardiovascular system examination and the paediatrician should carefully listen to the heart sounds and for heart murmurs. The first heart sound is caused by closure of the atrioventricular valves (mitral and tricuspid) and it is best heard at the apex, and the second heart sound is caused by closure of the aortic (first) and (second) pulmonary valves and it is best heard at the sides of the upper sternal edge.

Breathing will influence the closure of pulmonary and aortic valves and therefore usually change the character of the second heart sound. During inspiration the intra-thoracic pressure decreases leading to increased venous return to the right side (blood is pulled from the body into the vena cava by the negative intrathoracic pressure created by diaphragmatic descent) of the heart and reduced filling of the left side (the blood tends to stay in the lungs because of the vacuum surrounding the lungs) which delays the closure of the pulmonary valve relative to the aortic valve and results in a wider splitting of the second heart sound. In children with an atrial septal defect the flow of blood from left to right across the defective septum leads to a continuous increase in right atrial filling and therefore there is a wide and fixed splitting of the second heart sound which is independent of inspiration. It is louder in children with pulmonary hypertension as the pulmonary valve 'slams' shut.

A third heart sound, or gallop rhythm is often a sign of heart failure and is thought to be produced by rapid left ventricular filling, whereas a fourth heart sound occurs in conjunction with atrial contraction. The exact cause is not known but it may reflect increased atrial contraction. According to timing, murmurs are differentiated to systolic which can be ejection or pansystolic, diastolic and continuous. To understand the pathophysiology behind heart murmurs it is useful to remember the cardiac cycle.

This is divided into three basic stages: 1. Ventricle contraction, 2. Ventricle relaxation, 3. Ventricular filling. In the early contraction phase the pressure in the left ventricle increases until it exceeds the pressure in the left atrium then the mitral valve closes creating the 1st component of the 1st sound. Similar events happen on the right side but to a lesser magnitude creating the 2nd component (tricuspid) of the 1st sound. Because both mitral and aortic valves are closed, the left ventricle volume is fixed and the contraction is called isovolumic. The pressure in the left ventricle continues to increase and when it exceeds that in the aorta, the aortic valve opens. When the pressure in the aorta exceeds that in the left ventricle, the aortic valve closes creating the 1st component of the 2nd heart sound. Similar events happen on the right side resulting in the 2nd component (pulmonary) of the 2nd heart sound. As the pressure in the left ventricle falls to below that in the left atrium, the mitral valve opens and the left ventricle filling stage of the cardiac cycle starts.

Ejection clicks, result from stenotic aortic or pulmonary valves or dilated ascending aorta or pulmonary artery so they are heard in early systole. Pansystolic murmurs, are heard throughout systole and because they are heard during the ejection phase as well as the isovolumic phase during which both the atrioventricular valves and the aortic and pulmonary valves are closed, they must be caused by an insufficient atrioventricular valve or an abnormal opening like a ventricular septal defect. Continuous murmurs, are heard through systole and diastole, they result from a continuous blood flow through an aortopulmonary communication like a patent ductus arteriosus. Diastolic murmurs, are heard after the 2nd heart sound and before the 1st heart sound, so they are caused by either an insufficient aortic or pulmonary valve or a stenotic atrioventricular valve.

The Electrocardiogram (ECG) in evaluation of congenital heart disease

The electrical activity of the heart can be recorded using electrodes placed on the chest wall and limbs. The sinoatrial node is the pacemaker of the heart and initiates atrial depolarisation. After a short delay in the atrioventricular node, the electrical activity or the impulse is transmitted to the ventricles via His-Purkinje system. The sinoatrial node is located high in the wall of the right atrium and it produces P wave (atrial depolarisation) on the ECG. The P-R interval is the time between the onset of P wave (atrial depolarisation) and the onset of QRS complex (ventricular depolarisation). The QRS complex reflects the rapid ventricular depolarisation (ventricular activation) and happens as a result of the electrical activity traveling through the His-Purkinje system. The left side of the septum is activated first and then the right. The ST segment is the segment between the J point (end of QRS complex and ventricular depolarisation) and the beginning of T wave (beginning of ventricular repolarisation). The T wave represents ventricular repolarisation.

There are six chest leads (V1 to V6) and six limb leads (I, II, III, aVR, aVL and aVF). Leads II,III and aVF view the inferior surface of the heart, and V1-V4 view the anterior surface, while I, aVL V5 and V6 view the lateral surface. If the electrical wave travels towards a specific electrode; this will produce a positive or upright deflection and if the wave travels away from the electrode this will produce a negative or downward deflection. The cardiac axis refers to the direction of the ventricular depolarisation wave in the frontal plane. The normal axis is between -30 and 90. Any axis beyond -30 is called left axis and any axis >90 is called right axis.

Right atrial enlargement causes tall (peaked) P wave, while left atrial enlargement causes wide and prolonged P wave. Right ventricular hypertrophy on the ECG is reflected by dominant R wave in lead V1 and right axis deviation and left ventricular hypertrophy is reflected by tall R wave in the chest leads (more than 26mm in V4,V5 or V6), or the sum of R wave in V1 plus S wave in V5 or V6 is more than 35mm.

Syllabus Mapping

Cardiology

* know the anatomy of the commoner types of congenital heart disease
* understand how the anatomy of the heart relates to changes in physical signs including what underlies the heart sounds and murmurs
* understand how the electrical activity of the heart translates to the ECG
* be able to select and interpret appropriate investigations in a child with suspected cardiac pathologies

References and Further Reading

1. Bernstein D, Chapter 417-420 The cardiovascular system. Kliegman RM, Stanton BMD, Geme J et al. Nelson Textbook of Paediatrics. 19th ed. Philadelphia, Elsevier Saunders; 2011.

2. Veasy LG, Chapter 192, Cardiac Auscultation. Finberg L, Kleinman RE et al. Saunders Manual of Paediatric Practice. 2nd ed. Philadelphia, Pennsylvania. W.B. Saunders Company; 2002.

3. Meek S, Morris F, Chapter I, II, Leads, rate, rhythm, and cardiac axis. Basic terminology. Morris F, Edhouse J, Brady W, Camm J et al. ABC of Clinical Electrocardiography. BMJ Publishing Group; 2003.

4. Opie LH, Chapter 12, Mechanisms of Cardiac Contraction and Relaxation. Braunwald et al. Heart Disease A Textbook of Cardiovascular System. 5th ed. Philadelphia, Pennsylvania, W.B. Saunders Company;1997.

Chapter 7: The child with an irregular heart beat
Dr Conrad Bosman

Case 1: A 13 year old boy was brought to A&E after his first episode of syncope whilst playing football. His QTc was 560 milliseconds. This is a segment of his ECG:

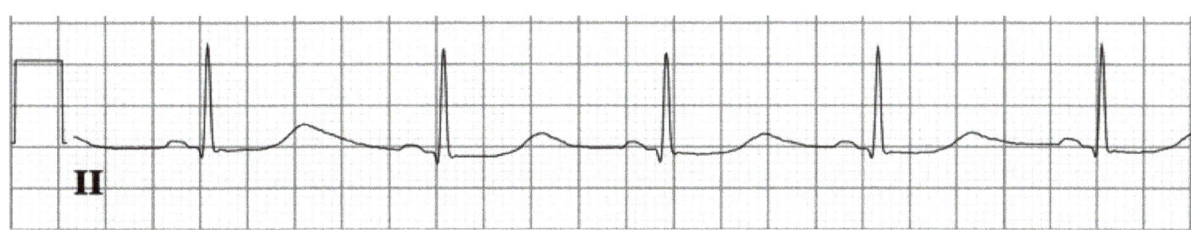

Case 2: A 15-year old girl was seen in clinic with recurrent fainting episodes in the morning when her alarm went off. Her QTc was 500 milliseconds. This is a segment of her ECG:

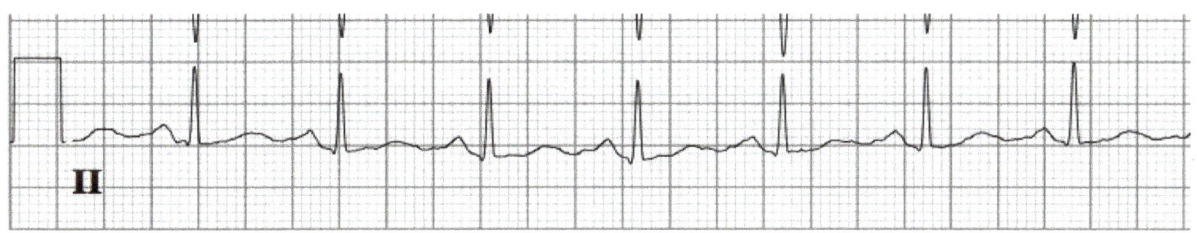

Case 3: An 8-year-old girl is seen in clinic. Her 25-year-old uncle died suddenly in his sleep. His post-mortem examination was normal. Her QTc was 490 milliseconds. This is her ECG:

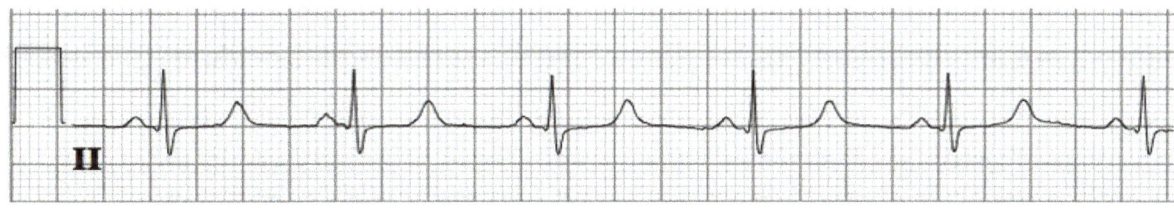

Q1.   What is the most likely cause of the prolonged QT segment in all of these cases?

A.   Romano-Ward syndrome
B.   Congenital channelopathy
C.   Jervel and Lange-Nielson syndrome
D.   Hypocalcaemia
E.   Hypokalaemia

Q2.   Which ion channel is most likely to be affected in case 1?

A.   The calcium channel
B.   The chloride channel
C.   The magnesium channel
D.   The potassium channel
E.   The sodium channel

Answer and Rationale

Q1.   Congenital channelopathy
Q2.   The potassium channel

Cases 1-3 are examples, respectively, of the first three types of congenital Long QT syndromes (LQT1, LQT2 & LQT3) (1). Each type corresponds to a different mutation in a gene responsible for a component of a cardiomyocyte ion channel and results in different patterns of late ventricular repolarisation. Note carefully the different T wave morphologies. See if you can describe them yourself before reading on.

Modern electrocardiogram (ECG) machines calculate both the QT interval and the QTc for you, the latter being the heart rate corrected QT interval. It is good practice, however, to manually calculate these parameters. Lead II in the rhythm strip is best, but alternatively leads V5 or V6 should be used. The QT interval is the time in seconds from the beginning of the Q wave (beginning of the first downward deflection of the QRS complex) to the end of the T wave (the point where the T wave returns to baseline). Standard ECGs are run at 25.0 mm/sec on graph paper where 1 mm (one little square) corresponds to 0.04 (1/25) seconds. Multiplying little squares by 0.04 gives the time interval in seconds.

A QT or QTc interval must be referenced with age and sex appropriate normograms, but generally any value above 480 ms is usually abnormal. Bazette's formula is commonly used to calculate the QTc (2) (Note: intervals for both QT and RR here must be in seconds, not milliseconds):

$$QTc = \frac{QT}{\sqrt{RR}}$$

Ventricular repolarisation involves the outward flow of potassium, and the inward flow of sodium and calcium through a complex system of ion channels in the cardiomyocyte. Any cause of a delay in the potassium extrusion, or a speeding up of sodium or calcium influx causes a prolonged QT interval. These causes can be congenital or acquired.

Congenital prolonged QT syndrome results from abnormalities in the ion channels, and contributes to 10% of cases of sudden unexpected death syndrome in infancy (SUDI). There are over 12 gene mutations that cause prolonged QT (1). The first three account for 99% of cases.

LQT1 is caused by a defect in the KCNQ1 gene at chromosome 11p15.5. It is the most common cardiac channelopathy, and slows potassium ion channels. The KCNQ1 gene also codes for a potassium ion channel in the auditory system and explains the link with congenital deafness. It causes a broad based and prominent T wave. Homozygotes for defects in the KCNQ1 gene are those first described by Jervell and Lange-Nielsen in 1957. The main precipitating factor towards ventricular arrhythmia is vigorous physical exercise, such as sprinting or swimming.

LQT2 (KCNH2 gene at chromosome 7q35-36) also slows cardiac potassium ion channels and causes a flatter (low amplitude) T wave. The T wave can also be notched. Arrhythmias are most commonly precipitated by emotional stress, such as a fright from an unexpected loud noise. LQT3 (SCN5A at chromosome 3p21-24) affects cardiac sodium ion channels, speeding them up. It causes a late onset (prolonged isoelectric ST segment), peaked (high voltage) T wave. Arrhythmias are most commonly precipitated during sleep or rest. Defects in these two genes as well as others were those originally described as being inherited via autosomal dominant inheritance by Romano (1963) and Ward (1964).

Acquired long QT syndrome is the result of any non-genetic factor that prolongs cardiac repolarisation. Main groups include drugs, electrolyte imbalance (hypokalaemia, hypocalcaemia, hypomagnesaemia and hyponatraemia), starvation / anorexia nervosa, metabolic and neurological conditions.

Syllabus Mapping

Cardiology

- understand how the electrical activity of the heart translates to the ECG
- be able to select and interpret appropriate investigations in a child with suspected cardiac pathologies
- know the genetic and environmental factors in the aetiology of heart disease
- know the physiological basis of myocardial function
- understand the pathophysiology of cardiac conditions including syncope and unexpected cardiac death
- know the possible cardiac complications of other system disorders

References and Further Reading

1. Modell SM, Lehmann MH. The long QT syndrome family of cardiac ion channelopathies: a HuGE review. *Genet Med* 2006;**8**:143–55.

2. Hunter JD, Sharma P, Rathi S. Long QT *syndrome. Contin Educ Anaesth Crit Care Pain* 2008;**8(2)**:67-70.

Chapter 8: Yet another blue baby
Dr Rana Alia

A 5 day old baby girl arrives in the emergency department having collapsed at home. She was born at 40 weeks gestation by an emergency Caesarean section for failure to progress. The mother had a febrile illness during the first trimester which was followed by poorly controlled gestational diabetes. Her birth weight was 2.4 Kg. Further history from mum reveals that over the past few hours the baby struggled to feed.

Q1.   Regarding the differential diagnosis for this baby's collapse, which of the following statements are true (T) or false (F)?

A.   Congenital cytomegalovirus infection significantly increases the risk of cardiac defects
B.   Congenital rubella infection leads to cardiac defects in more than 25% of those affected
C.   Elevated fetal insulin results in macrosomia and neonatal hypoglycaemia
D.   Growth restriction confirms that an infant is unaffected by maternal diabetes
E.   Ventricular septal defect is the commonest cardiac complication of gestational diabetes

Following resuscitation the infant is breathing spontaneously in 100% oxygen. Her heart rate is 170 beats per minute, respiratory rate 60 per minute, blood pressure 50/24 mmHg and oxygen saturation is 60% in the left foot. She has been started on Prostaglandin E1 infusion.

Q2.   Which ONE of the following statements is most correct?

A.   Impalpable femoral pulses confirm coaractation of the aorta
B.   Prostaglandin E1 infusion at recommended dose leads to apnoea in more than half of cases
C.   Prostaglandin E1 infusion is life saving in total anomalous pulmonary venous connection
D.   Prostaglandin E1 will result in increased blood pressure secondary to vasoconstriction
E.   Severe pulmonary stenosis is a duct dependent cardiac lesion

Answers and Rationale

Q1. **A. False**   **B. True**   **C. True**   **D. False**   **E. False**
Q2. **E. Severe pulmonary stenosis is a duct dependent cardiac lesion**

The fetal microenvironment has important consequences for the health of the newborn child. In turn this is dependent upon placental function and maternal health. Disruptions to normal maternal physiology may be well tolerated in the mother and potentially asymptomatic. Nonetheless, they can have severe consequences for the fetus.

Infant of the diabetic mother

Gestational diabetes mellitus is a disorder of carbohydrate metabolism which involves 2-5% of pregnancies in England and Wales. Congenital anomalies are 2-4 times more common in pregnancies complicated by diabetes. Treatment seems to reduce the risk of serious perinatal complications (1). Gestational diabetes has long term effects on the fetus and has been shown to be an independent risk factor for the development of ADHD (2).

Glucose is readily transferred across the placenta. Therefore, maternal hyperglycaemia is usually accompanied by fetal hyperglycaemia. This in turn leads to hyperinsulinaemia and hyperplasia of the pancreatic islet B cells. The elevated insulin leads to increased fetal growth of all organ systems except the brain. The macrosomia which is typical of infants of diabetic mothers can only occur if nutrients can be delivered in excess by the placenta. Therefore a child born to a pregnancy complicated by placental dysfunction of any cause will still be growth restricted. This child is paradoxically at greatest risk of hypoglycaemia in the newborn period as it will lack the reserves of larger infants.

Relative hyperinsulinaemia persists after birth. The sudden interruption of the glucose supply at birth typically results in early onset hypoglycaemia. However, insulin levels will typically fall rapidly after birth and hypoglycaemia beyond the first week should prompt investigation of other causes (MCAD, LCHAD). Babies with hypoglycaemia may be asymptomatic or they may display some non specific symptoms and signs like jitteriness, hypotonia, poor suck, tachypnoea, seizures and coma.

Cardiac anomalies are common in these infants occurring at a rate 10 times higher than that seen in other newborns (3). The most common abnormalities are cardiomegaly and asymmetry of the ventricular septum. Other morbidities which are more common in these infants include tachypnoea and surfactant deficiency, polycythaemia, jaundice, sacral agenesis, renal vein thrombosis, neural tube defect and small left colon syndrome. Infants of diabetic mothers are at higher risk of being obese and developing diabetes later in life. They also have an increased incidence of intellectual impairment.

The common manifestations of congenital infections (4)

The child described in our case is unexpectedly small. Intrauterine growth restriction is a common consequence of congenital infection and this should be considered as a possible cause. Many relatively common viral and bacterial infections have the potential to cross the placenta leading to teratogenetic effects. Varicella zoster virus, Rubella virus, Cytomegalovirus (CMV) and Toxoplasma gondii are the commonest seen in the UK although congenital syphilis, once consigned to a footnote within textbooks is beginning to occur more frequently. All these infections have the potential to cross the placenta during pregnancy and to cause congenital infections more commonly following a primary infection.

Rubella: If acquired in the first trimester, congenital anomalies can occur in over 80% of fetuses. Maternal infection between 13 and 16 weeks leads to deafness in about a third. Infection beyond 18 weeks is of little risk to either mother or child. Congenital rubella presents as a progressive disease and some abnormalities are not clinically evident at birth. Congenital rubella infection typically causes cardiac abnormalities like patent ductus arteriosus which is most common and occurs in about 30% of affected infants, pulmonary artery stenosis and pulmonary arterial hypoplasia also occur. Eye involvement causes cataract, retinopathy, microphthalmos and iris hypoplasia. Other manifestations include microcephaly, mental retardation, speech and language delay and hearing loss.

Congenital Varicella infection: Almost 15% of pregnant women are susceptible to varicella (Chickenpox). In most instances the fetus is unaffected but there are two 'at risk' periods. Maternal exposure to chickenpox in the first half of pregnancy leads to an approximately 2% risk of severe scarring of the skin, digital dysplasia and ocular or neurological damage. If a mother is infected with chickenpox shortly before delivery then the fetus is unprotected by maternal antibodies and the viral dose can be very high. This leads to a very severe infection and mortality in untreated babies is up to 30%.

Cytomegalovirus: CMV is the most common congenital infection affecting up to 1 in 250 live births in the UK. Almost 50% of pregnant women are susceptible to CMV and 1% of these will have a primary infection during pregnancy. In 40% of cases the infant becomes infected. 90% of infected infants are normal at birth and develop normally. Of the 10% who develop sequelae then approximately half have features at birth (hepatosplenamegaly, petechiae, jaundice growth restriction and occasionally seizures) whilst half develop problems later in life, mainly sensorineural hearing loss.

Toxoplasma gondii infection: is caused by a protozoan parasite. It can be acquired from consumption of raw or undercooked meat and from contact with the faeces of recently infected cats. It is rare in the UK and affects only about 1 in 10,000 live births. Most infected infants are asymptomatic. Of the 10% that show clinical features, the most common are chorioretinitis, cerebral calcification and hydrocephalus. Asymptomatic infants remain at risk of developing late-onset chorioretinitis. When a diagnosis is made then prolonged treatment with pyrimethamine, sulfadiazine and folic acid is recommended.

Duct dependent congenital cardiac disease

A number of congenital heart defects are dependent on the patency of the duct in order to maintain survival of the infant. These can be divided into those that are dependent on the duct for adequate pulmonary blood flow and those that required the duct to maintain systemic circulation. In both groups commencement of a prostaglandin infusion can be life-saving.

Ductal dependent pulmonary blood flow:
- Critical pulmonary stenosis
- Pulmonary atresia
- Tricuspid atresia with pulmonary stenosis/atresia

Ductal dependent systemic blood flow:
- Coarctation of the aorta
- Hypoplastic left heart syndrome
- Interrupted aortic arc

Whilst the classic presentation of coarctation of the aorta is with absent femoral pulses, in reality they can still be felt in some cases. Ordinarily the blood pressure in the lower limbs is approximately 10mmHg higher than in the arms. This is due to the direct transmission of pressure from the aorta to the larger descending aorta. The pressure is transmitted from aorta to the upper limb through a comparatively narrow vessel.   Coarctation of the aorta is suspected when the systolic pressure is 20mmHg lower in the legs than in the arms (5). Femoral pulses will be reduced in all cases of reduced cardiac output.

Prostaglandin E1 and E2
Prostaglandin E1 (alprostadil) and E2 (dinprostone) are vasodilators which maintain duct patency. As a side effect, cardiovascular events including hypotension, flushing and bradycardia are most common and occur in about 18% of infants. Apnoeas happen in about 12% of patients and are more likely to happen in infants less than 2 Kg.

Syllabus Mapping

Cardiology

- know the genetic and environmental factors in the etiology of heart disease
- understand the development of the heart and know the abnormalities that are associated with the congenital heart diseases
- know the anatomy of the commoner types of congenital heart disease
- understand the pharmacology of drugs used to treat common cardiac conditions including duct dependant cyanosis

Genetics

- know the environmental factors which may affect prenatal development

References

1. Crowther CA et al. Effect of treatment on gestational diabetes mellitus on pregnancy outcomes. *N Engl J Med* 2005;**352**:2477-2486

2. Nomura Y et al. Exposure to gestational diabetes mellitus and low socioeconomic status. Effects on neurocognitive development and risk of ADHD. *Arch Pediatr Adolesc Med* 2012;**166(4)**: 337-343.

3. Hornberger LK. Maternal diabetes and the fetal heart. *Heart* 2006;**92(8)**:1019–1021.

4. Chapter 9. Perinatal medicine. Illustrated textbook of paediatrics (4th Edition). Lissauer T and Clayden G. Elsevier, London 2012.

5. Tulloh R. Paediatric Mastercourse (2nd Edition) (in press).

Chapter 9: A boy with eczema
Dr Ian Petransky

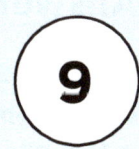

A 4 year old is sitting outside the clinic room waiting to be seen, he is scratching at his excoriated arms and you can see that his skin is lichenified.   He is keeping his family up at night due to scratching and being generally uncomfortable. He is attending for follow up review after an admission for eczema herpeticum. His brother is an inpatient on the ward with asthma, eczema and icythyosis vulgaris.

Q1. Concerning these children: which ONE of the following statements is the most accurate?

A.   Children with eczema have thickened skin which reduces permeability
B.   Ensuring a dry, cold environment in the home will alleviate the eczema
C.   Reduced barrier function of the skin predisposes to infection
D.   Reduced immune activity in eczematous skin increases the risk of infection
E.   Tacrolimus blocks calcium dependent proteases decreasing keratin turnover

The skin is a complex organ, intra and extracellular proteins interplay to support skin function. Match the protein/organelle from the list (A-J) with its described function:

A.   Actin
B.   Collagen
C.   Desmosome
D.   Dyenin
E.   Filaggrin
F.   Fibrin
G.   Hemi desmosome
H.   Keratin
I.   Troponin
J.   Tubulin

Q2.   Attachment to the basement membrane

Q3.   Destroyed in Staphylococcal scalded skin syndrome

Q4.   Hygroscopic to maintain water content of skin

Q5.   Main constituent of cytoskeleton in stratum corneum

Answers and Rationale

Q1. C. Reduced barrier function of the skin predisposes to infection

Q2. G. Hemi-desmosome   Q3. C. Desmosome

Q4. E. Filaggrin   Q5. H. Keratin

To answer the questions knowledge of how the mechanical and molecular barrier functions of skin are maintained is essential. This knowledge is useful as it helps us understand why we use different treatments and suggests a logical order in which those treatments should be used. The main function of skin is to act as a barrier. This barrier function promotes defence against pathogens, chemicals, temperature, humidity and ionising radiation. Skin also has immunological function, endocrine function (especially vitamin D) and even contributes slightly to gas exchange (1) (see also Chapter 10).

The skin is made up of the dermis and epidermis. The epidermis starts at the basement membrane and the cells of the epithelium divide and migrate from deep to superficial becoming more specialised as they move towards the surface. Each cell is bound to either the basement membrane by a hemidesmosome or to the surrounding cells by desmosomes.   Desmosomes are transmembrane proteins that are attached to the cytoskeleton of 'their' cell and linked to the desmosome of the adjacent cell. In this way every cell is directly bound to the cytoskeleton of adjacent cells and more distant cells. If desmosomes are broken down, as can occur with the toxins of Staphylococcal bacteria, skin shedding can occur with minimal trauma (Nikolsky's sign) (1,2).

Skin epithelium changes and becomes super-specialised as the cells migrate to the skin surface forming into a squamous shape (elongated flattened cells). This is achieved by filling of the cytoplasm with proteins especially keratin and cross linking these polymer fibres into strong stable networks. The squamous shape means the skin is resistant to mechanical trauma and allows shedding of skin without disruption of the whole surface (1-3).

Filaggrin is found in keratohyalin granules; these granules are present as the cells migrate from the prickle cell layer into the granular cell layer (stratum granulosum). It is within the granular cell layer that terminal differentiation occurs. The major constituents of the keratohyalin granules are keratin and profilaggrin, the promolecule of filaggrin. As the contents of the granules are released keratin forms long polymers called tonofilaments. Profilaggrin is also released from the granules and is broken down by the action of proteases to filaggrin. The filaggrin molecules cross-link the keratin tonofilaments. Cross-linked keratin provides the structural strength of the cornified cell layer on the outer most part of the skin. It is cross-linked keratin that forces the originally cuboidal epithelial cells into their squamous shape (1-3). The effects of filaggrin far outreach structural integrity of skin squames. It is directly involved in the moisturising actions of skin, antibacterial effect and possibly photoprotective effects (2,3).

Filaggrin is hygroscopic; it absorbs and holds onto water molecules becoming a hydrated molecule. As filaggrin is degraded by proteases amino acids are released which further add to the moisture retaining properties of the stratum corneum. The loss of water from these molecules is higher in dry environments and promotes filaggrin turnover. In warm humid environments there is less water loss from the hygroscopic molecules leading improved skin stability. Filaggrin and its degradation products, along with lipids present in the squamous cells, are referred to as natural moisturising factors.

Filaggrin degradation fulfils another important role. The resulting amino acids contribute to low skin pH, this 'acid mantle' suppresses bacterial growth and some of the degradation products have a direct anti-staphylococcal effect. Studies in filaggrin knockout mice show that the degradation products also contribute to protection of skin from ultraviolet radiation (2).

The most common skin conditions involving filaggrin are icthyoses and eczema. Both these conditions are exacerbated by cold dry weather. Icthyoses vulgaris (IV) is caused by loss-of-function mutations in the filaggrin gene. These are common in the general population and approximately 7.7% of Europeans and 3.0% of Asians have at least one filaggrin gene mutation. IV affects between 1:80 and 1:250 of the UK population. As well as cosmetic effects children with IV have an increased incidence of atopic eczema. Atopic eczema has an incidence of 10-20% in the developed world (2-4). Loss of function mutations in the filaggrin gene, lead to at least a three-fold increased risk of having atopic eczema. Filaggrin is the most common known gene defect associated with atopic eczema (4-6). Eczema herpeticum is also more likely in patients with filaggrin defects (7). Eczema treatments such as emollients and wet wraps increase the humidity close to the skin and boost its water-retaining qualities. This slows filaggrin degradation and leads to a significant clinical improvement in eczema.

Breakdown in barrier function for any reason leads to increased absorption of substances across the skin, easier passage of microbes through the skin and increased water losses from the skin. Skin can then become dry and itchy with more rapid shedding of squames from the stratum corneum giving the observed clinical picture in eczema and icthyoses. Loss of the acid mantle and structural integrity allows invasion of the skin by microorganisms and can lead to infection. Other substances are also more likely to traverse the outer layer of the skin and can then come into direct contact with the immune system. This is the mechanism by which eczema can lead to allergic sensitisation. Once a naïve immune system is exposed to new allergens immunological memory can be formed, after this repeated exposure will lead to inflammatory response (2,3). The inflammatory response caused by absorbed allergens also leads to the clinical picture of eczema. Once inflammation has occurred immunoregulators such as steroids and calcineurin inhibitors (tacrolimus) may be needed to relieve symptoms (8).

If skin barrier function can be optimised then hypothetically subsequent atopy may be avoided, infections decreased, and skin integrity maintained. Atopic conditions such as allergic rhinitis and asthma are associated with filaggrin gene defects especially if eczema is present (6). There is a UK study (Barrier Enhancement Eczema Prevention, BEEP study) at present (2013) that is looking to see if early emollients prevent atopic dermatitis occurring (9). It is conceivable that in the near future clinicians will encourage the use of emollients in at risk children to prevent the onset asthma and allergy. Simple treatments, such as the application of moisturisers, supports the longevity of filaggrin and its breakdown products conferring a myriad of short and long term benefits.

Syllabus Mapping

Dermatology

- understand the anatomy of the skin
- know how abnormalities in skin anatomy and physiology relate to appearance, dysfunction and disease
- understand the pharmacology of agents used to treat common skin diseases

References

1. Gardiner M, Eisen S, Murphy C. Training in Paediatrics the Essential Curriculum. Oxford University Press 2009. pp. 194-207.

2. Sadilands A, McLean WH. Filaggrin in the frontline: Role in skin barrier function and disease. *J Cell Sci* 2009;**122**:1285-1294.

3. Brown SJ, McLean WH. One Remarkable Molecule: Filaggrin. *J Invest Dermatol* 2012;**132**:751-762.

4. Irvine AD, McLean WH. Breaking the (un)sound barrier: filaggrin is a major gene for atopic dermatitis. *J Invest Dermatol* 2006;**126**:1200-1202.

5. Baurecht H, Weidinger S. Towards a major risk factor for atopic eczema: Meta-analysis of filaggrin polymorphism data. *JACI* 2007:**120(6)**:1406-1412.

6. Van den Oord R, Sheikh A. Filaggrin gene defects and risk of developing allergic sensitisation and allergic disorders: systematic review and meta-analysis. *BMJ* 2009;**339**:2433.

7. Gao PS, et al. Filaggrin mutations that confer risk of atopic dermatitis confer greater risk for eczema herpeticum. *JACI* 2009;**124**:507-13.

8. http://emedicine.medscape.com/article/911574 (accessed 29/09/2013)

9. http://www.beepstudy.org (accessed 29/09/2013)

Chapter 10: The child with a blistering rash
Dr Samundeeswari Deepak

A 9 month old boy, presents with blisters over his neck and left upper arm which appeared abruptly and have persisted over the last week. Initially these lesions are pink patches. These evolve over 48 hours to become blisters. Older lesions heal with crusting but without scarring.

Q1.   In which layer of the skin is pathology occurring?

A.   Dermis
B.   Dermal-epidermal junction
C.   Epidermis
D.   Subcutaneous
E.   Throughout dermis and epidermis

The following is a list of the layers of the skin:

A.   Basal cell layer (stratum basale)
B.   Dermoepidermal junction
C.   Granular cell layer (stratum granulosum)
D.   Horny layer (stratum corneum)
E.   Lamina lucidum (stratum lucidum)
F.   Papillary dermis
G.   Prickle cell layer (stratum spinosum)

Match the following conditions to the skin layer:

Q2.   Dystrophic epidermolysis bullosa

Q3.   Epidermolysis bullosa simplex

Q4.   Pemphigus vulgaris

Q5.   Staphylococcal scalded skin syndrome

Q6.   Toxic epidermal necrosis

Answers and Rationale

Q1. C. Epidermis **Q2. B. Dermoepidermal junction** **Q 3. A. Basal cell layer**
Q4. G. Prickle cell layer **Q5. C. Granular cell layer** **Q 6. B. Dermoepidermal junction**

The following table lists some of the commoner blistering skin conditions. They are placed in order of the skin layers which they predominantly affect starting with the most superficial:

Skin Condition	Clinical features	Pathogenesis	Scarring	Treatment
Bullous impetigo (1)	Vesicles, bullae	*Staph. aureus* infection. Exfoliative toxin mediated. Confined to the site of infection	No	Antibiotics-topical/ systemic
Staphylococcal scalded skin syndrome (1,2)	Macular erythema, sandpaper like rash, systemic features may be present	Epidermolytic toxin produced by *Staph sp.* act at a remote site leading to separation of superficial epidermis	No	Systemic antibiotics
Pemphigus foliaceus (1)	Superficial fragile blisters-easy to break (intraepidermal)	Autoantibodies against desmoglein 1 protein leading to disruption of superficial epidermal intercellular junctions	No	Immune suppression
Epidermolysis bullosa simplex (3)	Generalised blister with little systemic involvement	Inherited mainly autosomal dominant, rarely autosomal recessive. Cytolysis causes intraepidermal skin separation in the basal/spinous layer	No	Supportive
Pemphigus vulgaris (1)	Fragile blisters-easy to break (intraepidermal)	Autoantibodies against desmoglein 3 protein leading to disruption of deeper epidermal intercellular junctions	No	Immune suppression
Junctional EB (3)	Generalised blister with mucosal involvement: eyes, pharynx, GI tract	Autosomal recessive inheritance. Affects the dermal-epidermal junction	Variable	Multidisciplinary care
Toxic epidermal necrolysis (4)	Widespread erythema exfoliation, bullae & mucosal involvement leading to sepsis and death	Idiosyncratic reaction to infection medication or malignancy leads to apoptotic keratinocyte cell death in the epidermis with bullae formation due to dermal-epidermal separation	Yes	Supportive treatment Prevention of secondary infection Wound care
Dystrophic EB (3)	Generalised blister, mucosal involvement and systemic features	Autosomal dominant or recessive inheritance. Skin separation below the dermoepidermal junction.	Yes	Multidisciplinary care
Pemphigoid	Deep tense rigid blisters that do not break easily	Autoantibodies against basement membrane of epidermis lead to subepidermal blistering	Yes	Immune suppression

The skin is a bilayer organ composed of epidermis and dermis, which provide many protective functions essential for survival. The skin constitutes almost 1/6 of total body weight. It has four major functions: 1. Protection – against ultraviolet light, mechanical, thermal and chemical insults. It also has a relatively impermeable surface, which prevents dehydration and acts as a physical barrier to invasion by microorganisms; 2. Sensation; 3. Thermoregulation – the body is insulated against heat loss by the presence of hairs and subcutaneous adipose tissue. Heat loss is facilitated by the evaporation of sweat from the skin surface and increased blood flow through the rich vascular network of the dermis; 4. Metabolic functions as a triglyceride store and vitamin D synthesis.

The epidermis is composed of an outer layer of dead cells and keratin, which present a barrier to bacterial and environmental toxins. The epidermis has four or five layers, beginning with the outermost these are the: 1. stratum corneum, 2. stratum lucidum (only palms and soles), 3. stratum granulosum, 4. stratum spinosum and 5. basal cell layer. The cells in these layers (keratinocytes) are held together by organelles called desmosomes. Desmosomes are cell adhesion structures that are especially prominent in the epidermis and mucous membranes. The basal cell layer is the source of new epidermal cells, and rete pegs ensure attachment of the dermis to the epidermis via the basement membrane. Damage to the epidermis alone leads to blister formation but usually heals without scarring whilst damage to the dermal layer or epidermal-dermal junction leads to scarring.

The epidermis is supported and nourished by a thick layer of dense, fibro-elastic tissue called the dermis, which is vascular and contains sensory receptors. The dermis is attached to the underlying tissues by a layer of loose tissue called the hypodermis or subcutaneous layer, which contains variable amounts of adipose tissues.

There are 3 major blistering diseases which affect the epidermal skin layer: bullous impetigo, Staphylococcal scalded-skin syndrome and pemphigus. Although the causes of these conditions are very different, the underlying mechanisms overlap and account for some of the apparent clinical similarities seen between these rather different diseases (1). Staphylococcal skin infections are among the most common skin diseases in children. The blisters in bullous impetigo and the scalded-skin syndrome are both caused by exfoliative toxin released by Staphylococcus. There are two major serotypes of this toxin, A and B. Type A is produced and acts locally and results in bullous impetigo, whilst type B toxin circulates throughout the body, causing blisters at sites distant from the infection. Both forms of the toxin appear to act upon a desmosomal protein desmoglein 1. Both toxins cause intra- epidermal cleavage in the very superficial layers of the epidermis. In these regions the major cell adhesion molecule is desmoglein 1 (1). All types of Staphylococcal infections are most commonly seen in newborns, infants and young children as immunity is less well developed. Usually the lesions begin as vesicles that rapidly enlarge to form flaccid bullae. Lesions may vary from few localised to numerous widely scattered with little or no surrounding erythema. A pathognomonic finding of bullous impetigo is a ring of scale at the periphery of eroded lesion with a varnished surface. Staphylococci are isolated from the skin lesions of bullous impetigo whilst these are sterile in Staphylococcal scalded skin syndrome. The diagnosis is usually made clinically and can be confirmed by the culture of the aspirate from the lesion.

Pemphigus foliaceus and pemphigus vulgaris are autoimmune disorders which result from the production of IgG autoantibodies to desmoglein 1 and desmoglein 3 respectively. The former results in superficial blistering but the latter affects deeper layers of the epidermis (stratum spinosum) and mucous membranes as in these regions there is much more desmoglein 3 expression and much less desmoglein 1.

Syllabus Mapping

Dermatology

*   understand the anatomy of the skin
*   know how abnormalities in skin anatomy and physiology relate to appearance, dysfunction and disease
*   understand how injuries to the skin, including burns affect function
*   understand the role of infective agents in skin disease

References

1. Stanley JR, Amagai M. Pemphigus, bullous impetigo and the Staphylococcal scalded-skin syndrome. N Engl J Med 2006;**355**:1800-10.

2. Ladhani S, Evans RW. Staphylococcal scalded skin syndrome. *Arch Dis Child* 1998;**78**:85-88.

3. Fine JD. Inherited epidermolysis bullosa: recent basic and clinical advances. *Curr Opin Pediatr* 2010;**22(4)**:453-8.

4. Becker DS. Toxic epidermal necrolysis. *Lancet* 1998;**351**:1417-20.

Chapter 11: The infant with a burn
Dr Gisela Robinson

A 9 month old boy, Archie, attends the emergency department by ambulance with an 8cm x 3cm burn to the top of his right thigh. Both mum and Archie are extremely upset. The paramedics tell you that on arrival to the house mum was holding the infants leg under the cold tap. En route they had covered the wound with Clingfilm. Mum tells you she had fallen asleep with Archie in her bed, and woke to find Archie crying hysterically having rolled into the small gap between the radiator and the bed. When she extricated him she noticed a burn to his leg and so put it under the tap.

Archie is given some intranasal diamorphine, and the burn is examined. He has an oval burn running down the lateral aspect of his left leg, from just below his nappy line to the knee. Within it are 2 long fluid filled blisters with surrounding erythema. The blister is deroofed, the burn is dressed and Archie seems much happier.

Q1.   Which one of the following statements is correct? Select ONE answer only.

A.   Cellular skin damage occurs once the skin temperature reaches 45°C
B.   Contact burns cause more serious injury than scalds
C.   Destruction of rete pegs in the epidermis has led to blistering
D.   The zone of coagulation is the least likely part of the burn to become infected
E.   Thermal inertia is provided by the Meisseners corpuscles in the skin

Q2.   When considering if a burn is deliberate, which one of the following is true.

A.   Burns of varying depths are suspicious
B.   Child protection evidence is limited due to a paucity of published literature
C.   Childhood burns are rare, and need a joint medical with police and social care
D.   Most intentional burns are scalds
E.   The battered child was first described in the 1950s

Answers and Rationale

Q1.   C. Destruction of the rete pegs in the epidermis has led to blistering

Q2.   D. Most intentional burns are scalds

Burns occur at all ages but toddlers are at highest risk and highest overall rate of burn injury due to the combination of increasing mobility, curiosity and lack of life experience. This risk is amplified if motor skills development outpaces cognitive development. Understanding a burn injury requires an understanding of the anatomy and physiology of the skin. This has been discussed in detail in chapter 9 and 10. Loss of skin through thermal injury leads to functional impairment and can result in infection, hypothermia or water loss acutely and sensory deficits or scarring in the longer term.

The severity of a burn depends on burn depth, size, location and patient age, with infants and the elderly having highest mortality rates. The depth of heat injury depends on the degree of heat exposure and the depth of heat penetration. Wet heat (scald) travels more rapidly into tissue than dry (flame) heat because water conducts heat 100 times more efficiently than air. In addition skin thickness is crucial, the thinner the skin the deeper the burn will be. It takes only quarter of the time for a child to sustain a scald compared to an adult (1).

Contact with hot objects is the second most commonly occurring burn mechanism in small children (after scalds which are the cause in 66%(2)). When a hot object touches the skin the equilibrium temperature is dependent on the thermal inertia of both the object and the skin. Thermal inertia is related to the thermal conductivity, density, specific heat and the original temperature differences between the two. Cellular skin damage occurs once the temperature is greater than 49°C. Contact burns are usually small and to occur require the object to either be very hot – unlikely in a domestic radiator, or for contact time to be abnormally long (3) – this might occur if child was trapped between an object and a radiator for a period of time. The normal reaction to a painful stimulus is withdrawal, which limits the contact time in most situations.

Burn depth is anatomically defined by how much of the skin surface is destroyed. Burns are rarely of uniform depth throughout. Indeed a burn that was uniform in shape and depth would raise concerns of being caused by non-accidental injury: -

Superficial burn – confined to outer epidermal layer e.g. sunburn

Partial-thickness burn – involves epidermis and part of the inner dermis.

These are further subdivided into:

Superficial partial thickness – destruction of the entire epidermis and no more than the upper third of the dermis. The microvessels perfusing this area are injured, leading to leakage of large amounts of plasma. This lifts off the heat-destroyed epidermis and causes a blister to form. These are the most painful burns as the nerve endings are exposed to air. They look pink and wet.

Deep partial thickness burn – involves destruction of most of the dermal layer with few viable epidermal cells remaining. Blisters do not tend to form as the dead tissue layer is thick and adheres to the underlying viable dermis.   They are white and dry, but do have sensation – though pain is reduced as many nerve endings have been destroyed.

Full thickness burn – involves destruction of both dermis and epidermis, leaving no residual epidermal cells to repopulate. They are painless.

Subdermal burn – involves destruction of both layers and extends into the tissues below, including fat, tendons, muscle and bone.

Thermal injury to tissue is described in 3 zones. The area of superficial injury is the zone of hyperaemia and is warm and red. The middle area is the zone of stasis where the microcirculation is damaged and changes in capillary permeability allow fluids to leak from the vascular system into the interstitial space. The deepest area is the zone of coagulation where heat damaged cells occlude blood vessels, this obstruction in the microcirculation prevents the humoral components of the immune response from reaching the burned tissue. Transference of heat by a liquid results in a greater zone of stasis. This zone will evolve over the first 72 hours resulting in a more significant injury than on first assessment. This potential for 'continuing burn' has to be taken into consideration when managing scald injuries.

Severe burns are reported in an estimated 10-12% of children who have suffered from physical abuse, and burns and scalds are amongst the commonest causes of fatal child abuse. In addition a far greater number of accidental burns occur as a consequence of poor parenting decisions or neglect. Child protection literature has been around since the first published descriptive article on neglect and abuse in 1860 (4) the definition of the 'battered child' did not occur until the 1960's (5). Although interpretation of the evidence base concerning burn injury and child protection is difficult this is not because there are few published data. There are >16000 citations for child abuse in Pubmed, however using these data to draw conclusions about an individual case require experience and care. There are increasingly useful good systematic reviews being published by the Cardiff Child Protection Systematic Reviews (www.core-info. cf.ac.uk). These include information on the features that define accidental versus non accidental scalds, and proposing a triage tool to distinguish between them (6).

Syllabus Mapping

This question links to the syllabus under three headings:

Dermatology

*   understand the anatomy of the skin
*   understand how injuries to the skin including burns affect function

Pharmacology, Poisoning and Accidents

*   understand the epidemiology and psychosocial links of accidents in children

The Science of Practice

*   understand the principles of evidence based medicine and its limitations

References

1. Dresssler DP, Hozid JL. Thermal injury and child abuse: the medical evidence dilemma. *J Burn Care Rehabil* 2001;**22(2)**:180-5.

2. Drago DA. Kitchen Scalds and thermal burns in children 5 years and younger. *Pediatrics* 2005;**115(1)**:10-6.

3. Datubo-Brown D, Gowar JP. Contact burns in children. *Burns* 1989:**15(5)**:285-286.

4. Tardieu A. Etude medico-legale sur les services et mauvais traitements exerces sur les enfants. *Annales d'Hygiene Publique et Medecin Legale.* 1860;**13**:361-98.

5. Kempe CH, et al. The battered child syndrome. *JAMA* 1962;**181(1)**:17-24.

6. Maguire S, *et al.* A systematic review of the features that indicate intentional scalds in children. *Burns* 2008;**34**:1072-1081.

Chapter 12: The child with short stature
Dr Philippa Prentice, Dr Rachel Williams

Jessica is a 3 year old girl referred to the endocrine clinic with short stature. She was born at a normal birth weight (3.2 Kg) and length (49 cm). Her parents remember her always being shorter than other children. Measurements, which have been plotted in the hand-held 'red book' record, show that she has been growing with reducing growth velocity. Her current height of 84cm is currently well below the 0.4th centile (-2.9 standard deviation score), whilst her mid-parental height is on the 50th centile. On examination she has low muscle bulk and increased subcutaneous fat.

Q1. Which ONE of these tests would be LEAST useful in investigating Jessica's short stature?

A.   Bone age
B.   Karyotype
C.   Random serum growth hormone
D.   Serum IGF-1 and IGF-BP3
E.   Thyroid function tests

Q2. What would you expect to see on a hand radiograph, taken for assessment of bone age?

A.   Advanced bone age >1 year
B.   Delayed bone age >1 year
C.   Delayed bone age with shortness of 4th and 5th metacarpals
D.   Normal bone age
E.   Not appropriate to do a bone age

Answers and Rationale

Q1.   C. Random serum growth hormone

Q2.   B. Delayed bone age >1 year

Short stature is a common paediatric clinical presentation and has a wide differential diagnosis, for which the most common causes are shown below in table 12.1. The workup for short stature must always begin with a history and general investigations for exclusion of underlying chronic disease (eg malnutrition, renal disease or asthma), possible neglect, or other endocrine disease such as hypothyroidism (1). A karyotype should be done for all girls to exclude Turner's syndrome. A bone age is often very helpful.

Table 12.1 Main causes of short stature

Category	Cause
Genetic	Turner's Syndrome (Karyotype: 45 XO)
	Short stature homeobox gene (SHOX)
	Prader Willi Syndrome
	Trisomy 21 (and other Trisomies)
	Russell Silver Syndrome (Maternal uniparental disomy of chromosome 7)
Skeletal dysplasias	Achondroplasia/ Hypochondroplasia eg Fibroblast growth factor receptor 3 (FGFR3) mutations
Environmental	Intrauterine growth retardation
	Neglect
	Malnutrition
Chronic Illness	Inflammatory bowel disease, coeliac, chronic renal failure, liver disease
Iatrogenic	High dose inhaled/ systemic steroids
	Methylphenidate
Endocrine	Hypothyroidism
	Isolated Growth Hormone Deficiencies eg. GH1, GHRHR & SOX3 gene mutations/acquired/idiopathic
	Multiple pituitary hormone deficiency eg PROP-1 & POU1F1 gene mutations
	IGF-1 deficiency eg IGF-1 / IGF-1R gene mutations
	Cushing's Syndrome
	Hypoparathyroidism
Other	Familial short stature
	Constitutional growth delay

Growth hormone deficiency (GHD) is a relatively common endocrinopathy with an incidence of approximately 1 in 4000 (2). Most frequently it occurs as an isolated idiopathic GHD, with no cause found but may be part of a multiple pituitary hormone deficiency, or acquired for example due to a brain tumour so neuroimaging is always needed when a diagnosis is made.

Since GH does not affect intrauterine growth, birth measurements and early infancy growth are often normal. Early growth is mainly nutritionally regulated, and mediated by the hormones insulin and insulin-like growth factors. GH then predominately regulates childhood growth, from after infancy to puberty, and depending on the severity of GH deficiency, GHD will present in early or mid childhood with reduced height velocity. This classical presentation of isolated idiopathic GHD differs from that of a multiple pituitary deficiency, which commonly presents with jaundice and hypoglycaemia in the newborn period.

Growth hormone (GH) is synthesized in the anterior pituitary gland. It is released in a pulsatile fashion and predominantly regulated by two hypothalamic hormones: growth hormone releasing hormone (GHRH) and somatastatin, which stimulate and inhibit production of GH respectively. Basal secretion of GH is low in the day, with maximal GH secretion occurring in the early part of the night. Other physiological stimuli for GH release include stress, fasting, vigorous exercise, and hypoglycaemia.

Due to the pulsatile nature of GH release random GH measurements are of little value and GH stimulation tests are required to confirm a diagnosis of GHD. These are conducted after an overnight fast, using standardized protocols and one of the following pharmacological agents: arginine, clonidine, glucagon, insulin or L-dopa (3). The insulin tolerance test is the 'gold standard' stimulation test in children over 5 years. Glucagon stimulation tests are also frequently performed in the UK.

At a cellular level GH binds to GH receptor dimers, stimulating intracellular kinase cascades and gene transcription. GH leads to increased production of insulin-like growth factor (IGF-1) and to a lesser extent insulin-like growth factor binding protein 3 (IGF-BP3). GH exerts its biological effects mainly via insulin-like growth factor-1 (IGF-1), occurring at bone (at the growth plate), liver, fat and muscle. IGF-1 also inhibits both GH and GHRH by negative feedback. IGF-1 circulates bound to IGF binding proteins, the majority being bound with IGF-BP3 and acid-labile subunit (ALS). The actions of IGF-1 include growth of bone, cartilage and connective tissue, stimulating protein synthesis, cell proliferation and lipolysis. The clinical findings in GHD are therefore seen due to the reduced physiological action of GH and IGF-1. Children with GHD may have low muscle bulk and increased subcutaneous fat, with mid-facial crowding and delayed dentition.

IGF-1 concentrations are affected by age, gender, pubertal status, nutrition, intercurrent illness, chronic disease and ethnicity, as well as by height and body composition. This explains why faltering growth is not uncommonly seen in chronic disease, malnutrition or neglect. In contrast to GH, IGF-1 levels in the circulation are much more constant and low levels of IGF-1 and IGFBP-3 may suggest GHD if no other causes can be found. IGF-1 and IGF-BP3 can have a role in screening for GHD and clinically these are often done before GH stimulation tests, although it is important to know that in addition to physiological variation, IGF-1 levels are assay dependent and differ by centre (4).

It is important to assess bone age in all children suspected to have GHD. Bone age is a measure of skeletal maturity, usually calculated by rating a number of epiphyseal centres in the wrist, which are seen on x-ray. This allows an estimate of 'biological' age, from the rate of ossification seen, which can then be compared to the chronological age. A radiograph of the left hand is normally used.

Bone age is delayed in children with GHD (5), as well as those with constitutional delay of growth, hypothyroidism, chronic illness and malnutrition. In prepubertal children with GHD bone age is delayed with a mean of 2±1 year at age 6-10 years. Bone age is advanced in conditions such as precocious puberty, excessive androgen production (eg in congenital adrenal hyperplasia) and hyperthyroidism. Bone age determination is variable and for this reason a bone age more than one year less or greater than chronological age is taken to be abnormal.

Syllabus Mapping

Diabetes and endocrinology

- understand the physiological basis of growth and puberty
- understand the basis of growth measurement and charting
- understand the genetic and environmental factors that influence growth & puberty
- understand the pathophysiological basis of endocrine diseases such as diabetes and disorders of the pituitary and adrenal glands
- understand the appropriate investigation of endocrine disease

References

1. Drake AJ, Kelnar CJH. The evaluation of growth and the identification of growth hormone deficiency. *Arch Dis Child Educ Pract Ed* 2006;**91**;ep61-67.

2. Brook's Clinical Pediatric Endocrinology 6th Edition. Edited by Brook C, Clayton P, Brown R. 2009.

3. Growth Hormone Research Society. Consensus guidelines for the diagnosis and treatment of growth hormone (GH) deficiency in childhood and adolescence. Summary statement of the GH research society. *J Clin Endocrinol Metab* 2000;**85(11)**:3990-3.

4. Peters CJ, Dattani MT. How to use insulin-like growth factor 1 (IGF1). *Arch Dis Child Educ Pract Ed* 2012;**97**;114-118.

5. Martin DD *et al.* The use of bone age in clinical practice – part 1. *Horm Res Paediatr* 2011;**76**:1-9.

Chapter 13: The remarkably tall child
Dr Dita Aswani

Emma, a 12 year old Caucasian girl, is referred by her GP to a general paediatric out-patient clinic for investigation into her tall stature. She has always been tall compared with her friends, but on her transition to a large secondary school, she has become distressed by her size. Her parents are concerned she is feigning illness to avoid going to school. There are no academic concerns and reported normal intellect.

On examination she is prepubertal (her Tanner staging is A1, B1, P1). Blood pressure is 108/67 mmHg. There are no dysmorphic features. Full systemic examination is unremarkable.

She visits the auxologist and has her height, sitting height, arm span and weight measured. Height 170cm (>99.6th centile), Weight 40 Kg (50-75th centile), BMI 13.8 Kg/m^2 (just above 2nd centile), sitting height 83cm (75th -91st centile), and arm span 169cm. Her mother's height is 190cm and father's height is 185cm.

Q1. What is the most likely cause of her tall stature?

A.   Constitutional tall stature
B.   Growth hormone secreting tumour
C.   Homocystinuria
D.   Marfan's syndrome
E.   McCune Albright Syndrome

Q2. What should you do next?

A.   Bone age
B.   Chromosomes
C.   Growth hormone suppression test
D.   IGF-1 level
E.   X-rays of the long bones

Answers and Rationale

Q1. A. Constitutional tall stature

Q2. A. Bone age

In evaluating any child with tall stature the important thing to determine is whether tall stature in an individual is a normal variant or represents an underlying growth disorder. A hypothesis can be gleaned from 4 initial screening questions and then from elements picked out in a thorough history and examination: 1. Is growth velocity normal?; 2. Is height within the expected genetic target range?; 3. Is the child obese?; 4. Is the child proportionate?

Increased height velocity without obesity suggests endrocrine causes including hyperthyroidism, growth hormone excess, congenital adrenal hyperplasia (see chapter 15) or precocious puberty. In our case, Emma is slim and prepubertal. She is described as having been tall for some time suggesting a normal growth velocity. Furthermore both parents are tall and her height falls within the target centile range. Her arm span is somewhat less than her standing height but her sitting height is within the normal range suggesting long legs. This is consistent with a pre-pubertal stature as a significant proportion of height gain in puberty is from spinal growth.

The new UK growth charts for 2-18 year olds include a familial height scale to predict adult height and mid-parental centile. If you do not have one of these new charts to hand you can calculate the mid-parental height by the traditional method:

Mid-parental height (cm) = [Dad's height + Mum's height]/2 + 7cm for boys, or minus 7cm for girls

This can be plotted on a growth chart at age 18 to give you the mid-parental centile and 8.5cm either side of this will give you the target centile range (3rd and 97th percentiles). Of course there are limitations in assuming that tall stature is constitutional as several heritable causes of tall stature are associated with medical problems. Features of Marfan's should also be looked for in any tall child with tall parents as the syndrome is inherited as an autosomal dominant trait. One of the key features is increased arm span compared to standing height, which Emma does not demonstrate.

In children without learning difficulties proportionally longer legs are seen in Marfan's syndrome or hypogonadism. For those with learning disabilities it is important to consider homocystinuria, or chromosomal abnormalities e.g. Klinefelters syndrome. Body proportions are normal but there are associated dysmorphic features in Sotos syndrome, Beckwith-Wiedeman and neurofibromatosis. Non-constitutional, non-dysmoprhic proportionate tall stature is seen in children with ACTH insensitivity, oestrogen insensitivity or androgen insensitivity syndrome, and if onset is from early life in those with primary hyperinsulinism. Obese children are often tall, but final adult height is often not increased and skeletal maturation is advanced. In the MRCPCH exams often a clue to the diagnosis is buried in the clinical history a table of history and examination findings in different types of tall stature is shown opposite.

Key points	Diagnoses to consider
History of growth pattern Was it normal in infancy? When did period of accelerated growth start? Dietary history	Primary growth disorders (Sotos, Beckwith Wiedemann and Marfan's) often have high birthweights/lengths Those with constitutional tall stature or neurofibromatosis often have normal birthweights/lengths and show accelerated growth in infancy Children with underlying endocrine disorders or obesity may show accelerated growth at any stage
Neonatal history: Previous neonatal death Hypoglycaemia/abdominal wall defect	Beckwith-Wiedemann syndrome Congenital adrenal hyperplasia (See chapter 15)
Developmental delay/learning difficulties	Homocystinuria, Klinefelter's, Sotos
Eye problems: Lens or retinal detachment Glaucoma. Visual impairment. Visual field defects/visual loss	Marfan's syndrome or homocystinuria Growth hormone secreting tumour, optic glioma Pituitary tumours
Epilepsy and/or thrombosis	Homocystinuria
Cardiac abnormalities/family history	Valve prolapsed and aortic root dissection or widening in Marfan's syndrome
Weight loss, fatigue, muscle weakness, palpitations, tremor, diarrhoea	Hyperthyroidism
Large head or facial dysmorphism	Sotos, neurofibromatosis, Beckwith-Wiedeman
Abnormal sitting height:height ratio	Long legs and short back in Marfan's, Klinefelter's and gonadotrophin deficiency. Back grows in puberty (1).
Abnormalities of puberty: Early puberty Gynaecomastia/microorchidism	Precocious puberty Klinefelter's syndrome
Skin signs : Malar flush Café-au-lait patches	Homocystinuria Neurofibromatosis
Skeletal abnormalities: Arachnodactyly, Lax or hyperextendible joints, pectus excavatum, kyphoscoliosis	Marfan's syndrome and Homocystinuria
Androgen excess: Clitoromegaly, pubic hair, acne, body odour (in isolation)	Congenital adrenal hyperplasia Adrenal tunour

Syndromes with an extra Y chromosome such as Klinefelters (46 XXY), 47XYY or 48XYYY lead to tall stature in childhood and adult life independently of the GH level, which is not raised. The tall stature seen in sex chromosome aneuploidy conditions is thought to be due to the short stature homeobox gene (SHOX gene – see also chapter 12). It is a gene on the X and Y chromosomes which leads to short stature if mutated or present in only one copy (eg Turner Syndrome 45XO). Extra copies of SHOX are thought to lead to tall stature (2).

A left hand and wrist X-ray is used to determine skeletal maturation. Although not a diagnostic investigation, it often may provide reassuring information about final height prediction. Children with constitutional tall stature may have an advanced bone age suggesting final adult height may be reached at an earlier age. An advanced bone age is seen in obesity, precocious puberty, congenital adrenal hyperplasia, isolated glucocorticoid deficiency, thyrotoxicosis and Sotos syndrome. In hypogonadism the bone age is delayed. This information can be used to decide whether medical intervention is necessary. For this girl, her tall stature is already having serious psychological consequences, and as she has not yet entered puberty, still has a long time to grow. Girls will more often be concerned about being taller on average than will boys. After discussions with the family about predicted adult height, height reduction therapy may be considered. This could be achieved by treatment with exogenous oestrogen, to bring forward puberty and reduce final adult height. There are side effects to consider of weight gain, headaches, acne, thromboembolic events, development of ovarian cysts and dysmenorrhoea. In a boy, testosterone administration could be considered (3).

Syllabus Mapping

Diabetes and Endocrinology
* understand the physiological basis of growth and puberty
* understand the basis of growth measurement and charting
* understand the genetic and environmental factors that influence growth and puberty

Nutrition
* understand the principles of body composition in children and its basic assessment eg weight, BMI
* know the constituents of a healthy diet at all ages including the breast and formula feeding in infancy

Genetics and Dysmorphology
* understand the scientific basis of genetic disorders and inheritance
* be able to construct a family tree and interpret patterns of inheritance
* understand the chromosomal and molecular basis of genetic disorders

Ophthalmology
* know how the structure of the eye relates to function
* know about the eye manifestations of common systemic and genetic diseases

References

1. Fredricks AM, *et al.* Nationwide age references for sitting height, leg length, and sitting height/height ratio and their diagnostic value for disproportionate growth disorders. *Arch Dis Child* 2005;**90**:807-812.

2. Verge CF, Mowat D. Overgrowth. *Arch Dis Child* 2010;**95**:458-463.

3. Weimann E, Bergmann S, Böhles HJ. Oestrogen treatment of constitutional tall stature: a risk-benefit ratio. *Arch Dis Child* 1998;**78**:148-151.

Chapter 14: A child with adrenal suppression
Dr Sarah Eisen

A 7 year old boy is seen in the emergency department with a one day history of fever, shortness of breath and general malaise. Of note, the boy also has a history of nephrotic syndrome, diagnosed six months ago. He is currently in remission, and takes a maintenance dose of prednisolone daily (his mother cannot remember how much), as well as a prophylactic dose of penicillin V.

He has no allergies, his immunisations are up to date, and he lives with his parents and younger brother. On examination, he was tachypnoeic, tachycardic and febrile. Oxygen saturations were 92% on room air. His blood pressure was noted to be borderline high. His urine was negative on dipstick. He was slightly cushingoid, with no oedema. Examination of his chest revealed signs of a left lobar consolidation, confirmed on chest X-ray.

Cardiovascular and abdominal examination was unremarkable. A diagnosis of left lower lobe pneumonia was made. He was admitted and started on intravenous antibiotics.

Q1. Which of the following best describes his likely endocrine status?

A.   High cortisol, high adrenocorticotropic hormone and high corticotropin releasing hormone
B.   High cortisol, high adrenocorticotropic hormone and low corticotropin releasing hormone
C.   High cortisol, low adrenocorticotropic hormone and low corticotropin releasing hormone
D.   Low cortisol, low adrenocorticortopic hormone and high corticotropin releasing hormone
E.   Low cortisol, low adrenocorticotropic hormone and low corticotropin releasing hormone

Q2. How should you manage his steroid dose during this admission from an endocrine point of view?

A.   Do nothing, as he has been taking the same dose for some time
B.   Double his steroid dose by the oral route
C.   Double his steroid dose by the intramuscular route
D.   Review his steroid dose and consider weaning over the next week
E.   Stop his steroids immediately, as he is at risk of severe infection due to immunosuppression

Answers and Rationale

Q1.   E. Low cortisol, low adrenocorticotropic hormone, low corticotropin releasing hormone
Q2.   B. Double his steroid dose by the oral route

This is a boy who is on long term steroid treatment for nephrotic syndrome and is presenting with an intercurrent illness. Although his steroid dose is not known, this boy has been treated for some time at a dose sufficient to cause cushingoid appearance. It is therefore reasonable to assume that he may be suffering from iatrogenic adrenal insufficiency secondary to long term high dose corticosteroid administration (1).

Normally, adrenal secretion of cortisol is regulated by the hypothalamo-pituitary axis (HPA). The hypothalamus secretes corticotropin releasing hormone (CRH), which stimulates release of adrenocorticotropin hormone (ACTH) from the anterior pituitary gland. ACTH in turn stimulates release of cortisol from the zona fasciculata of the adrenal gland. This endogenous cortisol exerts negative feedback on the secretion of CRH and ACTH.

Administration of high dose glucocorticoids for more than about a week results in suppression of the HPA, resulting in reduced synthesis and secretion of CRH and ACTH and consequent hypofunction of the adrenal cortex, with downregulation of the natural synthesis of endogenous glucocorticoids (2). He is therefore likely to have low ACTH and low cortisol levels. Long term administration of high dose glucocorticoids may lead to adrenal atrophy, and full recovery of the HPA may take several months even after cessation of treatment (so be aware of possible adrenal insufficiency in patients who have recently discontinued glucocorticoid treatment as well as in those who are still on treatment).

Cortisol performs a variety of functions, including countering the effects of insulin, and exerting influences on vascular function, the inflammatory response, cardiac/skeletal muscle and water excretion. In the normal individual, there is a prompt synthesis and secretion of cortisol with stress (e.g. in intercurrent illness, as in this case, or surgery) and secretion remains elevated for several days. In his state of adrenal suppression, this patient is unlikely to be able to mount an effective stress response. It is therefore important to be alert for symptoms and signs of adrenal insufficiency (anorexia, headache, malaise, lethargy, nausea, vomiting and hypotension). Infants may become hypoglycaemic.

In this case, the boy was not showing signs of clinical adrenal insufficiency at the time of examination. However, it is nonetheless important that exogenous glucocorticoids are provided to compensate for the potential failure of the patient to mount his own cortisol stress response. Standard practice is to double or treble the current steroid dose. In this case, as the boy is not vomiting, it is appropriate to prescribe the double steroid dose by the oral rather than intramuscular route. In the case of surgery, steroids may be provided by an intravenous infusion. It is also important to pay close attention to hydration, electrolyte balance and blood glucose.

It is important that families are educated regarding the risks of adrenal suppression and that healthcare professionals are aware of the patient's condition. Wearing a Medic Alert bracelet, carrying a steroid treatment card, and holding a paediatric passport are all useful strategies. Parents should also be trained in the intramuscular administration of hydrocortisone for use in emergencies.

Various strategies can be used to reduce the likelihood of iatrogenic adrenal insufficiency (3). In general, the shortest possible course of steroids at the lowest therapeutic dose should be prescribed. Dosage should be on alternate days if possible as this ameliorates most longer term side effects. Evening doses of glucocorticoids particularly tend to suppress the normal early morning surge of ACTH secretion, resulting in greater adrenal suppression. Whenever possible, it is better to give a single morning dose. Where possible, avoidance of systemic therapy may reduce HPA suppression, though it is important to be aware some degree of suppression occurs even with high dose inhaled (4) or nasal (5) administration.

When reducing or discontinuing a steroid course, it is important to taper steroid doses carefully and not withdraw suddenly in patients taking steroids for more than a three week period (and in some patients with a shorter course as well) (3). Abrupt withdrawal may lead to an Addisonian crisis. This weaning process may be over a few days, if the course was short, but may take weeks or months if the patient had been on long term treatment.

When discontinuing steroid therapy, it may be useful to monitor the recovery of the HPA. This may be achieved by the short synacthen (ACTH) test, which may be performed after a steroid weaning programme is completed. This test evaluates the ability of the adrenal cortex to produce cortisol after stimulation by synthetic ACTH. Cortisol levels are measured at baseline and then at 30 and 60 minutes after ACTH stimulation. The standard dose of ACTH is 250 micrograms, a supraphysiological dose. The use of physiological doses (e.g. 1 microgram)) may prove useful in identifying those patients with partial adrenal insufficiency, such as may occur with chronic steroid treatment, as adrenal glands which are only partially suppressed may still show a response to the supraphysiological, but not to the physiological dose (6). Tests to assess the adrenal response to CRH may also be useful.

These tests should be performed in the morning, as the cortisol response to synacthen stimulation may vary significantly through the day, due to the normal diurnal pattern of cortisol secretion. Cortisol levels peak in the early morning (approximately 8 am) and reach their nadir three to five hours after the onset of sleep. This diurnal variation is believed to be regulated by communication of light reception by the retina to the paired hypothalamic suprachiasmatic nuclei. ACTH secretion is also circadian.

Syllabus Mapping

- understand the anatomy, embryology and function of the important endocrine organs, e.g. brain, thyroid, parathyroid, pancreas, adrenals and gonads
- understand the pathophysiological basis of endocrine diseases such as diabetes and disorders of the pituitary and adrenal glands
- understand the pathophysiological basis of endocrine emergencies, including diabetic ketoacidosis, adrenal crisis, hypoglycaemia, hyperglycaemia
- understand the appropriate investigation of endocrine disease
- understand the pharmacological basis of treatment of endocrine disorders
- know the possible impact on endocrine organs of other system disorders and vice versa

References

1. Alves C, Robazzi TC, Mendona M. Withdrawal from glucocorticosteroid therapy: clinical practice recommendations. *J Pediatr* 2008;**84(3)**:192-202.

2. Krasner AS. Glucocorticoid-induced adrenal insufficiency. *JAMA* 1999;**282(7)**:671-6.

3. Medicines Control Agency, Committee on Safety in Medicines. Focus on Steroids. *Current Problems in Pharmacovigilance* 1998;**24**:5-10.

4. Molimard M, Girodet PO, Pollet C, Fourrier-Reglat A, Daveluy A, Haramburu F, Fayon M, Tabarin A. Inhaled corticosteroids and adrenal insufficiency: prevalence and clinical presentation. *Drug Saf* 2008;**31(9)**:769-74.

5. Gill G, Swift A, Jones A, Strain D, Weston P. Severe adrenal suppression by steroid nasal drops. *J R Soc Med.* 2001 July; **94(7)**:350–351.

6. Chrousos GP, Kino T, Charmandari E. Evaluation of the hypothalamic-pituitary-adrenal axis function in childhood and adolescence. *Neuroimmunomodulation* 2009; **16(5)**:272-83.

Chapter 15: The child with congenital adrenal hyperplasia
Dr Philippa Prentice, Dr Rachel Williams

Case 1

You assess Alfie, a 10 day old baby boy, who has become unwell over the last 24 to 36 hours. He was born at term, with no complications during pregnancy or delivery. He had been breast feeding well at home but has lost weight, been vomiting more frequently and become increasingly sleepy. He is pale, tachycardic and hypotensive.

Q1. Which of the following results of investigations would lead you to suspect a diagnosis of adrenal insufficiency, for example due to congenital adrenal hyperplasia?

	Sodium (mmol/L)	Potassium (mmol/L)	Glucose (mmol/L)
A.	122	2.1	1.9
B.	122	6.9	1.9
C.	155	2.1	1.9
D.	155	2.1	3.8
E.	122	6.9	3.8

[Normal ranges: Sodium 135-145, Potassium 3.5-5.0, Glucose 3.0-7.8]

Case 2

A baby is born with abnormal external genitalia, which you suspect to be very virilised female genitalia as there are no palpable gonads. Birth and antenatal history are unremarkable, and there is no significant family history. You know that congenital adrenal hyperplasia is a likely cause of such a presentation.

Q2. Which of the following are the most relevant immediate diagnostic tests?

A.   Karyotype and 17-OHP both sent after 72 hours
B.   Karyotype and 17-OHP both sent immediately
C.   Karyotype and imaging of the adrenal glands
D.   Karyotype and sequencing of the CYP21A2 gene
E.   Karyotype sent immediately followed by 17-OHP after 72 hours

Answers and Rationale

Q1. B. Sodium 122, Potassium 6.9, Glucose 1.9.

Q2. E. Karyotype sent immediately followed by 17-OHP after 72 hours

Congenital adrenal hyperplasia (CAH) constitutes a group of autosomal recessive disorders, with an incidence of roughly 1 in 15,000 (1). CAH is caused by a deficiency in one of the five enzymes needed for steroidogenesis – the pathway allowing biosynthesis of cortisol from cholesterol. In the vast majority of cases (>90%) this is 21-hydroxylase deficiency (2). Most patients are compound heterozygotes, with the severity of disease determined by the activity of the less severely affected allele.

The clinical features occur due to the inability to produce sufficient cortisol (hypoglycaemia and hypotension), and more variably the mineralocorticoid, aldosterone (hyponatraemia and hyperkalaemia), in addition to accumulation of steroid precursors (virilisation of females). Since there is a blockage in the steroid enzyme pathway, any steroid precursors above this block will accumulate, which is reflected by the blood, and related urinary steroid metabolite profiles.

21-hydroxylase converts progesterone to deoxycorticosterone (see figure 15.1) and 17-hydroxyprogesterone (17-OHP) to 11-deoxycortisol. 17-OHP and related metabolites accumulate in 21-hydroxylase deficiency. In excess these are converted to androgens, causing virilisation in girls. At the same time, there is a deficiency of cortisol and/or aldosterone (depending on residual enzyme activity). The pituitary hormone ACTH stimulates cortisol production from the adrenal gland and is itself regulated by negative feedback. In CAH, when there is a lack of this negative feedback, increased ACTH stimulation starting in fetal life, causes hyperplasia of the adrenal glands.

Depending on the enzyme affected, the presentation of CAH may differ. Clinical symptoms also vary due to the degree of enzyme deficiency and therefore 21-hydroxylase deficiency can present as a salt-wasting state in the neonatal period, or as a much milder phenotype, with virilisation in newborn girls, without salt loss. Another presentation is in early childhood with pubic hair growth (sometimes referred to as late-onset or non classical CAH).

Our two clinical cases are classic neonatal presentations. Alfie's presentation is typical of that seen for a male baby, generally presenting extremely unwell with adrenal insufficiency at 7-14 days of age. Lack of cortisol, a counter-regulatory, catabolic hormone, results in hypoglycaemia. Associated deficiency of the mineralocorticoid aldosterone results in hyperkalaemia, hyponatraemia and resultant hypotension, hence the term 'salt wasting crisis'. There are often no signs of CAH at birth, although there may be subtle hyperpigmentation and penile enlargement. The main important differential diagnoses are other causes of adrenal insufficiency, sepsis and secondary hypoaldosteronism (pseudohypoaldosteronism). Secondary hypoaldosteronism may occur as a result of urinary tract infection with aldosterone resistance possibly as result of endotoxin damage to the aldosterone receptors. This results in hyponatraemia, hyperkalaemia and metabolic acidosis but most frequently with normoglycaemia (3).

Girls are more likely to present as newborns with virilisation, but it is important not to miss this phenotype so that neonates do not re-present in adrenal crisis. It is therefore crucial to check for palpable gonads in any phenotypically 'male' baby.

Figure 15.1. The adrenal gland steroid pathway from cholesterol to cortisol, aldosterone and androstendione, highlighting some of the main enzymes involved.

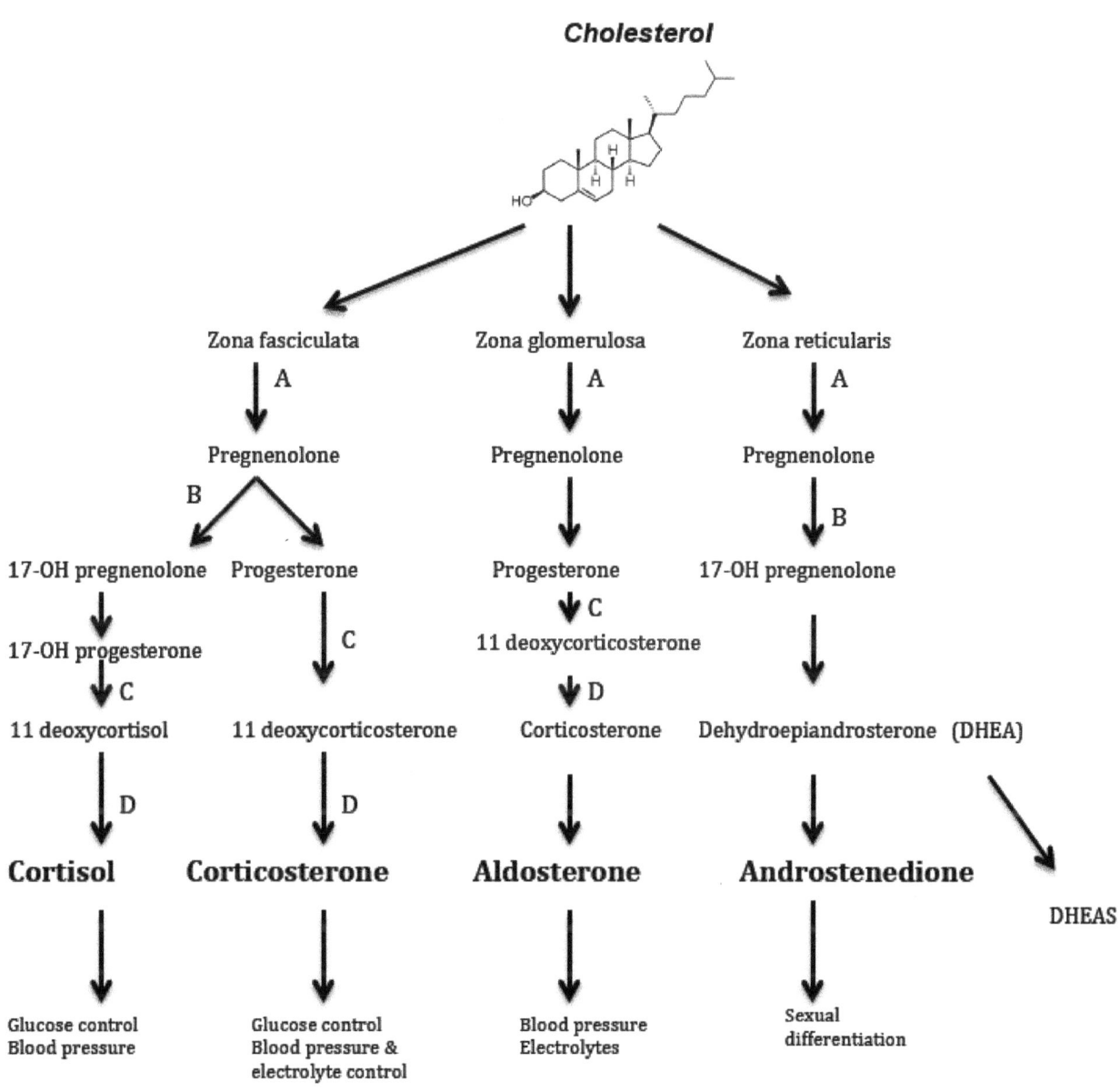

A Cholesterol side-chain cleavage enzyme (P450scc)
B 17 alpha-hydroxylase
C 21 hydroxylase
D 11 beta-hydroxylase

The diagnosis of CAH is made with a high random 17-hydroxyprogesterone (17-OHP). However, as the fetal adrenal is very metabolically active, 17-OHP and other adrenal metabolites are normally high in the fetus and the first few days of life and so the results can be difficult to interpret in the newborn period particularly in prematurity. Therefore, 17-OHP levels should only be taken after 72 hours of age and analysed urgently, so that the diagnosis is made promptly, before biochemical abnormalities or symptoms occur. It is also important to begin monitoring sodium, potassium and glucose at this stage, and to continue until a stable treatment regime has been initiated.

A confirmatory urinary steroid profile may also be helpful. For a newborn presenting with abnormal external genitalia other investigations may be needed, especially if the 17-OHP is normal. The most useful test whilst waiting for the 17-OHP is a karyotype.

The treatment of CAH is hormone replacement, with hydrocortisone and fludrocortisone (as needed) (4). Treatment of neonates with CAH is especially challenging as the electrolyte abnormalities are more difficult to correct, due to marked aldosterone resistance particularly during the first year of life which results in significant urinary salt loss, despite mineralocorticoid replacement. Infants may need treatment with salt, at doses which may seem very high in order to maintain normal electrolytes.

Syllabus Mapping

Diabetes and endocrinology

- understand the pathophysiological basis of endocrine diseases such as disorders of the pituitary and adrenal glands
- understand the pathophysiological basis of endocrine emergencies including adrenal crisis
- understand the appropriate investigation of endocrine disease

References

1. Speiser PW, White, PC. Congenital Adrenal Hyperplasia. *N Engl J Med* 2003;**349**:776-788.

2. Merke P, Bornstein S. Congenital adrenal hyperplasia. *Lancet* 2011;**365**:2125-36.

3. Peddle MB, Joubert G, Lim R. Case 2: Hyponatraemia and hyperkalemia in a four-week-old boy. *Paediatr Child Health* 2008;**13(5)**:387-390.

4. Hindmarsh PC. Management of the child with congenital adrenal hyperplasia. *Best Pract Res Clin Endocrinol Metab* 2008;**23(2)**:193-208.

Chapter 16: The Obese Child
Dr James Law

You are the registrar in a general paediatric clinic. You see a new patient referred by the GP because the school nurse has identified that they are overweight.

Below is a list of causes of obesity. Please select the most appropriate option for each case.

A.   Acquired hypothyroidism
B.   Albright hereditary osteodystrophy (pseudeohypothyroidism)
C.   Congenital hypothyroidism
D.   Cushing's disease
E.   Growth hormone (GH) deficiency
F.   Leptin deficiency
G.   Panhypopituitary dysfunction
H.   Prader-Willi syndrome
I.   Simple obesity
J.   Turner's syndrome

Q1.   A 10 year old girl whose weight plots 5 squares above the 99.6th centile and their height is on the 98th centile. Mum and dad are of a similar build. Mum is on thyroxine for acquired hypothyroidism. A food diary shows that she has cereal for breakfast, a packed lunch for lunch and a home cooked meal for tea and has no snack. The family explain she's always active and they can't understand why she doesn't seem to lose weight. On examination you notice some brown discolouration of her axilla, but the examination is otherwise unremarkable.

Q2.   A 6 year old boy whose weight is on the 99.6th centile and height is on the 25th centile. They were admitted to the neonatal unit postnatally due to some concerns regarding hypotonia. Initially they fed poorly and there were concerns about growth for the first couple of months. Just before being referred by their health visitor they started to gain weight and from 3 years old gained weight rapidly. Parents say they really struggle to stop him eating and he seems obsessed about food. On examination he appears to be a cheerful pleasant boy although parents tell you he can be very stubborn. You think his tone is slightly reduced.

Q3.   A 15 year old girl feels that over the last 6 to 12 months she has gained weight. She's gone from a size 10 to a size 14. Her weight is on the 98th and her height on the 75th. She thinks the weight gain is because she's not been doing as much exercise as previously as she doesn't feel she has as much energy which she's put down to the extra school work with GCSEs. However her school performance has also suffered recently. On examination she has a regular heart rate of 60 and you think you can feel a faecal mass in the left iliac fossa.

Answers and Rationale

Q1. **I. Simple obesity. Tall and normal examination make other causes unlikely. Overweight parents are a risk factor for obesity. The discolouration is acanthosis nigricans.**

Q2. **H. Prader-Willi Syndrome. Classic history of hypotonia from birth causing feeding problems initially followed by obesity in mid childhood associated with hyperphagia.**

Q3. **C. Acquired hypothyroidism. Change in rate of weight gain should alert you. Hypothyroidism is also associated with poor concentration, decreased energy, bradycardia and constipation.**

Obesity is caused by an imbalance between energy in (diet) and energy out (exercise/activity). Internationally rates of obesity are rising. Prevalence is highest in the Western world but the fastest rates of rise are in the developing world. In the UK, one third of 2-15 year olds are either overweight or obese including over a fifth of reception children. The percentage of overweight & obese 2-15 year olds has remained static since 2007. In children over 2, BMI is a useful measure of adiposity; BMI charts are available (overweight >85th centile for age and obese >95th). Under 2, weight may be a better indicator.

The aetiology of obesity is a mixture of environmental factors (activity levels and/or diet) acting on genetic predisposition – some individuals gain weight easily while others appear "resistant". The genetic influences are multifactorial and poorly defined apart from a few syndromic and monogenetic causes. In the paediatric clinic it is important to be able to recognise whether the obesity is a symptom of an underlying disorder or is due to a "simple" energy imbalance. The history, examination and growth chart will help to distinguish one from the other. Overweight children who are tall are much less likely to have an underlying cause. Obesity with onset under 2 years of age is more likely to be due to a syndromic cause. History and examination should ascertain details of any learning difficulties / developmental delay, dysmorphic features, abnormal tone, eye signs, hearing problems and cardiac abnormalities.

Obesity is associated with a reduced life expectancy and reduced quality of life. Children who are obese are more likely to go on to become obese adults.

- **Endocrine** complications include a spectrum from insulin resistance to type 2 diabetes mellitus, as well as polycystic ovarian syndrome and effects on growth.
- **Cardiac** complications include hypertension, dyslipidaemia, early stages of atherosclerosis and coronary heart disease.
- **Musculoskeletal** effects: slipped upper femoral epiphysis and Blount's disease.
- **Respiratory** complications include obstructive sleep apnoea.
- **Gastrointestinal** complications: gallstones and non-alcoholic fatty liver disease.
- **Psychological** increased incidence of depression, bullying and poor body image.
- **Neurological** complications include Idiopathic intracranial hypertension.
- **Dermatological** complications include striae and acanthosis nigricans.

	Growth	Genetics	Learning	Associations	Dysmorphism	Eyes
Acquired hypothyroidism	Excess weight gain with normal or slow height velocity	Usually sporadic	Poor school performance↓ ability to concentrate	Autoimmune or thyroid ablation. Usually high TSH, low T_3/T_4		If preceded by Grave's then signs may persist
Albright hereditary osteodystrophy	Small stature, moderate obesity	AD. Mutation in GNAS1 gene (subunit of G_s protein)	Average IQ of 60	↑PO_4 with ↓or↔Ca^{2+}. Variable mineralisation of tissues	Rounded face, short 4th and 5th metacarpals/ metatarsals	Cataracts
Alström Syndrome	Early childhood obesity	AR. ALMS1 gene mutation	Delayed milestones. Typically mild-moderate LD	Cardiomyopathy. Hearing loss. Liver /kidney problems. Insulin excess	Hypogonadism	Retinal dystrophy, photophobia nystagmus, strabismus
Bardet-Biedl Syndrome	Early childhood obesity; ht usually <50th centile	AR. Variable expression. Loci: 16q21, 11q and chr 3.	Moderate to mild LD. Odd mannerisms.	Kidney abnormalities, small penis/testes	Hypogonadism, polydactyly, syndactyly	Retinitis pigmentosa, cataract, strabismus
Carpenter Syndrome	Obesity; postnatal growth <25th percentile	AR. See with RAB23 gene defects (GTPase)	Variable from moderate LD to normal	Cardiac defects (50%), hypogenitalism, cryptorchidism	Acrocephaly, polydactyly, syndactyly, high arched palate	Coreneal opacity, optic atrophy.
Cohen Syndrome	IUGR, early poor growth with obesity from 5-6 years	AR. Mutations in VPS13B (aka COH1 gene)	Mild to moderate LD	Hypotonia and hypermobility. Delayed puberty. Cryptorchidism.	Microcephaly, prominent central incisors. Large ears.	Decreased visual acuity, strabismus.
Congenital hypothyroidism	Small stature and may be overweight	Usually sporadic but 2% is AR.	Delayed development (untreated)	Thyroid dysgenesis in (80%).	Rarely septo-optic dysplasia (SOD)	In SOD optic atrophy & nystagmus
Congenital or acquired GH deficiency	Usually normal at birth. Small stature with variable BMI.	Several genes identified:GH1, SOX2,SOX3, POU1F1.		Can be isolated or in association with other hypopituitary. If congenital, may be associated with neonatal hypoglycaemia.		
Hypothalamic / hypopituitary dysfunction	Short stature with obesity	Usually sporadic		Usually follow head trauma or tumours		May have bitemporal hemianopia
Leptin deficiency / Leptin receptor deficiency	Massive early obesity (from birth). Height usually normal	Severe forms are AR. OB gene (7q32).		Hyperphagia. Hypogonadotrophic hypogonadism, ↓TSH pulsatility, late puberty,↓adult height,↑bone age. ↑infection with ↓CD4/T-cell count.		
Prader-Willi Syndrome (see also chapter 21)	Faltering initially then obesity from 6 months	Imprinting. Absence of paternal copy of 15q11-13	Mild LD in 2/3rds, moderate in 1/3	Hypotonia. Excess appetite. Obsessive eating. Nasal speech	Thin upper lip. Almond-shaped palpebral fissure Hypogonadism.	Strabismus
ROHHAD	Rapid Onset obesity at 2-5yrs	Unknown		Hypothalamic dysfunction, Hypoventilation, and Autonomic Dysregulation. Neural crest tumours		Strabismus
Steroid excess	↑central obesity. Usually ↓ linear growth. Wasting of extremities	Usually sporadic. May be iatrogenic.	Learning can be affected and may not return to pre-treatment state	Moon face, buffalo hump, skin thinning, easy bruising, striae. ACTH dependent hyperpigmentation. ACTH dependent causes: Cushing's disease, ectopic ACTH/CRH. ACTH independent causes: Adrenal secretion, exogenous		All rare: Ex-opthalmos (retroorbital fat) Cataract ↑ intraocular pressure
Turner's syndrome	Small stature. Tendency to obesity.	XO. Mosaicism possible.	Mild LD and often delayed motor skills.	Streak ovaries. Kidney and cardiac defects.	Lymphoedema at birth. Shield chest. Webbed neck.	

The management of obesity is aimed at different levels: national policies, local implementation and individual management. On an individual level, management is aimed at increasing activity and improving dietary intake.

Syllabus Mapping

Diabetes and endocrinology

* understand the assessment, epidemiology and public health consequences of obesity

Nutrition

* understand the scientific basis of nutrition
* understand the principles of body composition in children and its basic assessment, eg weight, BMI
* know the possible nutritional consequences of being underweight and overweight on other body systems, eg cardiac and on long-term health
* know the epidemiology of obesity and malnutrition in global child health

References and Further Reading

1. Nelson Textbook of Pediatrics. 19th ed. Philadelphia, Elsevier Saunders; 2011

2. Smith's Recognizable Patterns of Human Malformation 5th Edition ISBN 0-7216-6115-7

3. Health Survey for England 2011 (http://www.ic.nhs.uk/catalogue/PUB09302)

4. WHO: Obesity (http://www.who.int/topics/obesity/en)

5. RCPCH growth charts (http://www.rcpch.ac.uk/child-health/research-projects/uk-who-growth-charts/uk-who-growth-charts)

6. National Obesity Observatory (http://www.noo.org.uk)

7. National Childhood Measurement Programme (http://www.hscic.gov.uk/catalogue/PUB09283)

Chapter 17: A baby with too little gut
Dr Asheeta Gupta

A 9 month old boy has been referred to clinic with faltering growth. He was born at 28 weeks gestation and spent two months on the NICU. During this time he was surgically treated for necrotising enterocolitis and underwent 2 laparotomies with bowel resections and subsequently has been given a diagnosis of short gut syndrome. He was initially on parenteral nutrition but has been on to a full enteral diet for the past month. You notice his weight has dropped from the 25th to less than 0.4th centile. His mother tells you he is taking his food and milk well with no vomiting. She notices that his abdomen looks distended at times but he seems well. He passes loose stool several times a day, which gets worse as he eats more and if she stops his feed the diarrhoea resolves.

On examination, he is afebrile and pale. His cardiorespiratory examination is normal. His abdomen is distended but there is no organomegaly and bowel sounds are present.

Q1. What is the most likely diagnosis?

A.   Bacterial overgrowth
B.   Infective diarrhoea
C.   Osmotic diarrhoea
D.   Secretory diarrhoea
E.   Toddler's diarrhoea

Q2. On reviewing his notes you see that he has had an extensive ileal resection. From the following list what specific problems is he at risk of developing?

Mark each stem as either True (T) or False (F).

A.   Gallstones
B.   Genu varum
C.   Oxalate stones
D.   Macrocytic anaemia
E.   Microcytic anaemia

Answers and Rationale

Q1. C. Osmotic diarrhoea

Q2. A. True   B. True   C. True   D. True   E. False

Short gut syndrome is a disorder of malabsorption caused by a congenital absence or extensive surgical resection of the small bowel. This question relates to the physiological functions of the duodenum, jejunum and ileum as well as the specific problems that can arise as a consequence of their absence.

Anatomically the duodenum and jejunum are distinct, but in terms of physiology they could be considered together as they perform similar functions. They act to promote further digestion of carbohydrate, fat and proteins by stimulating pancreatic enzymes, bile acids and production of brush border enzymes. The jejunum in particular is the main site of carbohydrate, protein, sodium and water absorption, which is all interlinked. Digested carbohydrates (galactose and glucose) and proteins (amino acids and tripeptides) are transported by coupled active transport together with sodium via the glucose sodium transporter 1 on the apical surface of the enterocyte. The exception to active transport is fructose, which moves down a concentration gradient by facilitated diffusion, which is an energy-independent method (1). The movement of solutes out of the intestinal lumen produces an osmotic gradient. The intestinal mucosa is a semi-permeable membrane with pores in the membrane at intercellular junctions. These pores allow passive movement of water along the osmotic gradient and electrochemical gradients created by actively transported solutes and sodium (2). The jejunum is more permeable to water than the ileum and therefore the majority of water absorption takes place here.

In short gut syndrome a number of factors disrupt solute and sodium absorption including: lack or dysfunction of digestive enzymes; reduced surface area; and intestinal hurry due to lack of the Diffuse Neuro-Endocrine Hormones (DNES) that act to reduce transit time (such as peptide YY which is produced in the ileum). This decrease in transit time is compounded by a lack of the ileocaecal valve, which acts as a physical barrier to delay small bowel emptying. These effects combine to disrupt the electrochemical and osmotic gradients needed for passive absorption of water provoking an osmotic diarrhoea. The diarrhoea stops if a patient stops eating.

Secretory diarrhoea occurs when the bowel mucosa produces excessive amounts of fluid due to activation of specific pathway by a toxin such as bile acid. Bile acids are normally mostly re-absorbed in the ileum. If this has been resected then bile acids may reach the colon in large quantities. Bacteria in the colon deconjugate the bile acid which stimulates chloride and hence water secretion into the bowel lumen leading to a secretory diarrhoea (3). Even if the patient stops eating the diarrhoea still continues.

Short gut syndrome can also cause a mixed osmotic and secretory diarrhoea caused by bacterial overgrowth, this is sometimes called an infective diarrhoea. The theory behind this is controversial but has been suggested to be due to absence of the ileocaecal valve resulting in colonic contents washing back into the ileum or jejunum. The bacteria can cause damage to the mucosa causing osmotic diarrhoea as well as stimulate secretory mechanisms in the colon to release water back into the bowel lumen resulting in a secretory diarrhoea (4). It presents with abdominal distension, foul-smelling stools, diarrhoea, flatulence, signs of vitamin B12 and fat soluble vitamin deficiency and systemic upset.

In this case the patient most likely has an osmotic diarrhoea as it resolves on stopping feeds. This is not an uncommon problem in short gut syndrome and is overcome by using parenteral nutrition to help growth of the child and slow introduction of enteral feeds to gradually allow the intestine to adapt to the loss of a particular section and take over its function. The ileum can take over function of the duodenum and jejunum and vice versa with the exception vitamin B12 and bile salt absorption, which are specific to the ileum.

Vitamin B12 is released from ingested proteins by pepsin in the stomach. It then binds to R-proteins to avoid degradation by stomach acid. Intrinsic factor (IF) is produced from parietal cells in response to the presence of food in the duodenum. Proteases in the duodenum digest R-proteins and release B12 which then binds to the IF. The B12/IF complex can then be absorbed in the terminal ileum by a specific receptor mediated channel. Vitamin B12 malabsorption results in a macrocytic anaemia. Longstanding depletion in vitamin B12 results in a demyelinating neuropathy leading to hypotonia, myoclonus and regression of development (5). The adverse effects of lack of fat soluble vitamins are summarized below (6).

Bile salts play a number of roles including aiding fat absorption. Fatty acids and monoglycerides (products of hydrolysed triglycerides) together with cholesterol and fat soluble vitamins are encased by bile salts and phospholipids in the duodenum and jejunum to form micelles. At the cell membrane the lipid contents of the micelles are absorbed while the bile salts remain in the lumen. Inside the cell the monoglycerides and fatty acids are re-esterified to triglycerides. The triglycerides and other fat soluble molecules are then incorporated into the chylomicrons to be transported into the lymph (1). Bile salts are not absorbed in the jejunum, so the intraluminal concentration in the upper gut is high. They pass down the intestine to be absorbed in the terminal ileum and are transported back to the liver. This enterohepatic circulation prevents excess loss of bile salts.

Ileal resection causes bile salt depletion due to malabsorption. This leads to fat and fat soluble vitamin malabsorption from inadequate micelle formation. There is a higher intraluminal concentration of fat, which binds calcium to form soap and prevents it from binding dietary oxalate. Rather than being excreted the oxalate is absorbed causing high plasma levels. This leads to steatorrhoea (fatty stools), fat soluble vitamin malabsorption (for effects see Table 17.1 below) and renal oxalate stones. Bile salt depletion can result in gallstones (cholelithiasis) as the remaining micelles become supersaturated with cholesterol. Cholesterol monohydrate crystals can precipitate out within the gallbladder and hence gallstones begin to form (1).

Table 17.1: Summary of the clinical effects of fat-soluble vitamin deficiencies (6)

Vitamin	Effects of deficiency
A	Night blindness, dry eyes, corneal opacification, Bitot spots (keratinisation of the cornea) Keratomalacia or hyperkeratosis Growth failure Immune dysfunction
D	Rickets (Growth retardation, tetany, muscle weakness, bone pain, skeletal deformities e.g. craniotabes, rachitic rosary, genu varum)
E	Neuroaxonal degeneration Progressive neuropathy Retinopathy
K	Deranged coagulation (Low prothrombin, factors VII, IX and X) Bleeding diasthesis

Syllabus Mapping

Gastroenterology and Hepatology

- know the anatomy and embryology of the gastrointestinal tract and how variation relates to specific disorders e.g. malrotation, atresias, Hirschprung's
- understand the anatomical and physiological and hormonal changes in gut and liver that occur throughout childhood
- understand the physiological basis of normal gut function including motility, absorption and secretion
- understand the role of the gut in homeostasis and its dysfunction

References

1. Kumar, P and Clark, ML. Gastrointestinal disease. *Clinical Medicine* (Eighth edition). Saunders (W.B.) Co Ltd; 8th Revised edition edition. 20 July 2012.

2. Whyte, LA and Jenkins, HR. Pathophysiology of diarrhoea. Occasional review. *Paediatrics and child health* 2012;**22(10)**:443-447.

3. Walters, JRF. Managing bile acid diarrhoea. *Therap Adv Gastroenterol* 2010;**3(6)**:349–357.

4. Kirsch, M. Bacterial Overgrowth. *Am J Gastroenterol* 1990;**3**:231-7.

5. Emery, ES. Vitamin B12 Deficiency: A Cause of Abnormal Movements in Infants. *Pediatrics* 1997;**99(2)**:255.

6. Blecker, U et al. Fat Soluble Vitamin Deficiencies. *Pediatrics In Review* 1999;**20(11)**:394-5.

Chapter 18: The child traveller with loose stool ⑱
Dr Simon Li

A 14 month old boy of Asian origin is referred to the paediatric assessment unit with a five week history of persistent diarrhoea. He has returned from India having been on holiday for two weeks visiting grandparents. On examination the patient was on the 0.4th centile for weight having previously been on the 25th centile. From a cardiorespiratory perspective he was stable. His abdomen was soft and non tender with no organomegaly. He was however considered to be 5% dehydrated and, in view of a failed fluid challenge, was made nil by mouth and started on intravenous fluids.

FBC was normal and his urea and electrolytes showed mildly elevated urea (8.6mmol/L). A stool sample was negative for reducing substances with the culture still pending. A urine dipstick was positive for ketones (++).

Over the course of the next 24 hours his diarrhoea abated. By the following morning he was able to tolerate dioralyte and by the afternoon had eaten half a slice of toast and yoghurt without any recurrence of symptoms. He was considered well enough by the evening to be discharged home but just as he is about to leave he suddenly gets severe and explosive diarrhoea.

Q1. What is the most likely diagnosis?

A.   Cholera infection
B.   Coeliac disease
C.   IgE-mediated cow's milk protein allergy
D.   Lactose intolerance
E.   Thyrotoxicosis

Q2. What should you do next?

A.   Advise switching to lactose free milk
B.   Arrange for allergy skin tests
C.   Perform testing for coeliac disease
D.   Screen for thyroid autoantibodies
E.   Send stool sample for viruses

Answers and Rationale

Q1. B. Coeliac disease
Q2. C. Perform testing for coeliac disease

The answer to this clinical case can be derived from an understanding of basic gut physiology and immunology. Firstly we need to consider the pathophysiology of diarrhoea which, in essence, is the imbalance between absorptive and secretory processes within the digestive tact. There are three major types of diarrhoea which are osmotic, secretory and motility disorders. Determining which type a child has is useful as it helps narrow the differential diagnosis. In osmotic causes of diarrhoea the mucosa of the intestine is often damaged and so absorption of osmotically active nutrients cannot take place. The unabsorbed nutrients create an osmotic gradient which draws water into the lumen of the intestine. If this exceeds the absorptive capacity of the gut then diarrhoea ensues. Such nutrients can be present for a variety of reasons such as malabsorption of specific solutes or damage to the absorptive area of the mucosa resulting in less fluid absorption. Secretory diarrhoea refers to the intestinal epithelial cells which are actively secreting ions and water into the lumen. This can be due to activation of specific pathways by toxins or be due to inherent abnormalities in the epithelial cells. Again if absorptive mechanisms are overwhelmed diarrhoea follows. Motility diarrhoea is caused by the reduction in the amount of time luminal contents have in contact with the bowel. Examples include patients who have had a vagotomy procedure or who have hyperthyroidism. The first clue in the question is the fact that the patient's diarrhoea resolved once enteral feeds were stopped which points to an osmotic cause. With no osmotically active solutes within the intestinal lumen the infant's diarrhoea settles and so we can immediately rule out cholera and thyrotoxicosis.

Lactose is a disaccharide comprised of the monosaccharides glucose and galactose. Absorption of lactose requires sufficient lactase to split lactose into its constituent parts. Testing for stool reducing substances is a simple and cost effective investigation which detects the presence of malabsorbed carbohydrates including lactose, fructose and galactose. Clinitest® is based on the ability of reducing substances present in stool to "reduce" the copper salts present within the reagent solution which is detected by a colour change. Given that testing for stool reducing substances is negative we can exclude lactose intolerance as the cause of the above case. It's also useful to get an idea of the stool pH as if it's less than 5.5 (i.e. acidic) it gives greater credence to a carbohydrate malabsorption problem, whether that be lactose intolerance or otherwise.

This leaves us with two options and to decide between the two we need to refer back to basic immunology. Food allergies can be divided into two types; those that are IgE mediated and those that are IgE independent. IgE-mediated food allergies are the type I hypersensitivity reactions as originally described by Gell & Coombs. This allergic reaction is predominantly driven by the formation of IgE antibodies which bind to mast cells. Subsequent mast cell degranulation and release of histamine causes an immediate reaction, with leukotriene release resulting in more delayed symptoms. Thus in IgE mediated cow's milk protein allergy we would expect an immediate reaction (typically within 30 minutes) upon ingestion of the food. Typical symptoms include abdominal pain, vomiting and diarrhoea. Non-intestinal symptoms include wheals, angioedema, wheezing and coughing. In its most severe form, anaphylaxis ensues and, in such instances, immediate administration of adrenaline is required to halt the inflammatory cascade.

Coeliac disease is a multifactorial disease where a genetic predisposition and environmental exposure are necessary. The disease is not IgE-mediated but is in fact considered a variant of type IV delayed hypersensitivity reactions arising from a cell-mediated response. The gliadin fractions of wheat gluten are the environmental factors responsible for the development of intestinal damage and symptomatology. Gluten peptides undergo deamidation by tissue transglutaminase (tTG) which creates immunostimulatory epitopes that bind to HLA-DQ2 or HLA-DQ8 on antigen presenting cells. This in turn activates CD4+ T-cells which secrete Th1 cytokines such as interferon-gamma resulting in enterocyte apoptosis and villous atrophy. CD4+ T-lymphocytes also produce Th2 cytokines which causes the activation and clonal expansion of B-lymphocytes. These in turn differentiate into plasma cells and produce antibodies against gluten and tissue transglutaminase which contributes to intestinal damage. This forms the basis of serological testing for coeliac disease by way of IgA tTG antibodies. A word of warning however – a significant proportion of coeliac sufferers have a low total IgA and in such cases it's necessary to look at the fraction of IgG tTG. The gold standard for diagnosis is however small bowel biopsy whilst on a gluten diet. Typical changes whilst on gluten include crypt hypertrophy, villous atrophy and intraepithelial lymphocytes. As the name suggests these reactions are typically delayed in onset and can occur anytime from a few hours up to days after ingestion of the offending food. In the case above his symptoms settled when made nil by mouth but returned a few hours after ingestion of toast. Hence the answer to the above case is coeliac disease and he requires a work up with a coeliac screen.

Syllabus Mapping

Gastroenterology and Hepatology

* know the basic histopathology and cellular dysfunction of important disorders including coeliac disease
* understand the physiological basis of normal gut and liver function including motility, absorption and secretion
* understand the role of the gut in homeostasis and its dysfunction
* know the genetic and environmental factors in the aetiology of gut and liver disease

Infection, Immunity and Allergy

* know the genetic and environmental factors in the aetiology of allergic and autoimmune disorders
* understand the scientific basis of atopy and anaphylaxis and the rationale for treatments

References

1. Saltzman W and Brown-Whitehorn TF. Gastrointestinal syndromes associated with food allergies. *Curr Probl Adolesc Care* 2012;**42**:164-190.

2. Lynch JP and Metz DC. Celiac disease: from pathogenesis to novel therapies. *Gastroenterology* 2009;**137**:1912-1933.

3. Whyte LA and Jenkins HR. Pathophysiology of diarrhoea. *Paediatr Child Health* 2012; **22 (10)**;443-447.

Chapter 19: The child with diarrhoea
Dr Mark Anderson

The following are causes of diarrhoea.

A. Cholera
B. Coeliac disease
C. Congenital glucose-galactose malabsorption
D. Cow's milk protein allergy
E. Crohn's disease
F. Giardia
G. Lactose intolerance
H. Laxative abuse
I. Shigella
J. Toddler's diarrhoea

Select the most likely cause from the list above that explains the following clinical scenarios:

Q1.   An 11 year old girl recently returned from Angola with large volume loose pale stools that persist even when nil by mouth

Q2.   A 3 week old boy with loose stools from 1-2 days of age which are now streaked with blood

Q3.   A 14 year old girl with chronic diarrhoea and weight loss and dark brown pigmentation of her colonic mucosa on colonoscopy.

Answers and Rationale

Q1. C. Cholera
Q2. D. Cow's milk protein allergy
Q3. H. Laxative abuse

Diarrhoea is a common presenting symptom to both acute and outpatient paediatric services, and is generally defined as having three or more loose or liquid stools per day. An understanding of the mechanism of causation of diarrhoea as well as the age at which the various causes present is useful in delineating aetiology.

The various mechanisms of diarrhoea are as follows:

- Osmotic diarrhoea occurs when water-soluble molecules are poorly absorbed from the intestinal lumen resulting in retention of water in the intestine. Osmotic diarrhoea stops with fasting.
- Secretory diarrhoea occurs as a consequence of an increase in the active secretion of fluid and electrolytes into the intestinal lumen and results in a significantly larger volume of liquid stool than osmotic diarrhoea, which persists in spite of fasting.
- Exudative diarrhoea occurs as a consequence of an alteration in membrane permeability and serum proteins, blood and/or mucus are exuded into the intestinal lumen. Stool volume is typically small.

Typically, disease processes have more than one mechanism resulting in diarrhoea, although one usually is preponderant.

In the first case of diarrhoea in a returning traveller, the key points are the large volume stools that persist even when fasting, suggesting a secretory cause. This is typical of the presentation of cholera, which is the commonest cause worldwide of secretory diarrhoea. The other two potential infective causes, Giardia and Shigella, typically cause exudative diarrhoea.

Cholera is caused by the bacterium Vibrio cholerae. It is transmitted by contaminated food or water and a significant number of bacteria must be ingested in order to cause cholera, although children aged 2-4 years and individuals with type O blood are most susceptible. The majority of ingested bacteria fail to survive the acidic conditions of the stomach, but those that reach the wall of the small intestine are able to reproduce and generate the toxin that is responsible for the secretory diarrhoea. Cholera toxin consists of six protein subunits – one A subunit and five B subunits. The B subunits bind to GM1 gangliosides on the surface of the intestinal epithelial cells resulting in internalization of the toxin by endocytosis. The A subunit then ADP-ribosylates the α-subunit of the heterotrimeric Gs protein leading to permanent activation. This results in constitutive production of intracellular cAMP and as a consequence the cystic fibrosis transmembrane conductance regulator is activated resulting in a dramatic efflux of electrolytes and water into the intestinal lumen and the appearance of so-called "rice-water" stools. (1)

In the second case of early onset diarrhoea in a young infant, the possible causes from those offered include lactose intolerance and congenital glucose-galactose malabsorption. However, neither of these results in the colitis suggested by the presence of blood in the stool, which is typical of non-IgE mediated cow's milk protein allergy. Non-IgE mediated cow's milk protein allergy was previously known as cow's milk protein intolerance, but its nomenclature has changed to reflect the immunological nature of the condition and to differentiate from the non-immunological lactose intolerance. The exact pathogenesis of allergic colitis is not clear but it has been proposed that a T-cell mediated mechanism causes intestinal cell damage. Colitis is more unusual in IgE-mediated cow's milk protein allergy. (2)

Lactose intolerance is caused by the absence or reduction of the enzyme lactase which is expressed exclusively in the enterocytes of the small intestine, predominantly in the brush border. Lactose cannot be directly absorbed. Lactase hydrolyses the disaccharide lactose into the monosaccharides glucose and galactose, which can be directly transported across the intestinal epithelium. In the absence of lactase, lactose passes into the colon where it is metabolized by bacteria resulting in fermentation products that cause osmotic diarrhoea. Congenital glucose-galactose malabsorption is an autosomal recessive condition resulting from a mutation in the gene encoding the sodium/glucose co transporter protein SGLT1. SGLT1 facilitates the uptake of glucose and galactose from the intestinal lumen. Its dysfunction results in osmotic diarrhoea by the same mechanism as absence of lactase, but glucose-galactose malabsorption results in life-threatening dehydration.

In the third case of diarrhoea in a teenager with weight loss, inflammatory bowel disease, in particular Crohn's disease, must be a prime consideration. However, the finding of dark brown pigmentation of the colonic mucosa at colonoscopy is typical of melanosis coli, most commonly caused by extended use of laxatives. Biopsy reveals pigment-laden macrophages. The brown pigment is lipofuscin, not melanin as the nomenclature would suggest. Anthraquinone containing laxatives, in particular senna, are the most likely culprits. Melanosis coli is a not uncommon finding at colonoscopy in adults. However, in the clinical case detailed here, an eating disorder must be suspected. (3)

The clinical presentation of coeliac disease and the science underpinning this are discussed in more detail in Chapter 18. Toddler's diarrhoea is the commonest cause of persistent loose stool in preschool children. The stool in these children is a variable consistency but the presence of undigested vegetables within the stool is common. There is probably more than one cause for toddler's diarrhoea but the child thrives and therefore malabsorption is not a feature. Increasing the fat content of the diet can improve the symptoms as dietary fat will slow the gut transit time.

Syllabus Mapping

Gastroenterology and Hepatology

- understand the physiological basis of normal gut and liver function, including motility, absorption and secretion
- know the genetic and environmental factors in the aetiology of gut and liver disease
- understand the pathophysiology of infective agents in the gut and liver

References

1. Muanprasat C, Chatsudthipong V. Cholera: pathophysiology and emerging therapeutic targets. *Future Med Chem* 2013;**5**:781-98.

2. Koletzko S *et al.* Diagnostic approach and management of cow's-milk protein allergy in infants and children: ESPGHAN GI Committee Practical Guidelines. *JPGN* 2012;**55**:221-229.

3. Roerig JL *et al.* Laxative abuse:epidemiology, diagnosis and management. *Drugs* 2010;**70**:1487-503.

Chapter 20: The baby with pale stools
Dr Ramani Gunasekera, Dr Will Carroll

A 16 day old baby is admitted to the ward with a 48 hour history of poor feeding, diarrhoea and vomiting. She was born at term weighing 3.2 Kg following a spontaneous vaginal delivery. She has been exclusively breast fed. Her weight on admission was 3.4 Kg. Since admission she had tolerated her feeds without vomiting and her diarrhoea is settling.

On examination she active and alert, pink and well perfused. Her mucous membranes are moist. She is jaundiced and her sclerae are greenish yellow in colour. Her abdomen is soft and non-tender and her liver is palpable 2.5cm below the costal margin. She has normal bowel sounds. She has just opened her bowels and her nappy contains a pale but otherwise normal looking stool. Mum explains that her stools have always been pale apart from the first few of days of life.

Q1. **What is the most likely cause for her jaundice?**

A.   Biliary atresia
B.   Breast milk jaundice
C.   Congenital cytomegalovirus infection
D.   Cystic fibrosis
E.   Hepatitis A

Q2. **What makes normal stool brown?**

A.   Caesin
B.   Hemosiderin
C.   Ligandin
D.   Lipase
E.   Stercobilin

Q3. **Breakdown of haemoglobin by the reticuloendothelial system can be determined by measurement of which exhaled gas?**

A.   Carbon dioxide
B.   Carbon monoxide
C.   Hydrogen
D.   Nitric oxide
E.   Nitrogen

Answers and Rationale

Q1. **A. Biliary atresia**
Q2. **E. Stercobilin**
Q3. **B. Carbon monoxide**

Pale stools in a jaundiced baby should always prompt consideration of biliary atresia. A thorough understanding of bilirubin metabolism is necessary to answer the type of questions encountered in both the MRCPCH Theory and Science exam and clinical practice.

Unconjugated bilirubin is the product of haem metabolism. Most haem metabolism is as the result of red blood cell breakdown. During the first few weeks of life there is a gradual reduction in red cells with a commensurate drop in blood haemoglobin concentrations as the newborn adjusts to extrauterine life. Each haem molecule will produce one molecule of bilirubin. These molecules are found in haemoglobin, myoglobin and cytochrome enzymes. The production of bilirubin from haem occurs mainly in the spleen (macrophages) and liver (Kupfer cells) but occurs throughout the body in macrophage and even in the renal tubular cells. The cells that perform this function form the reticuloendothelial system.

Red blood cell breakdown in the reticulo-endothelial system produces haem and globin molecules. Globin is broken down into amino acids. Haem is oxygenated releasing iron (which is recycled) and carbon monoxide and producing biliverdin which in turn is then reduced to form the antioxidant bilirubin. Unconjugated bilirubin is carried in the circulation as a complex bound to albumin. At lower levels this binding prevents diffusion into either the urine or peripheral tissues. This unconjugated bilirubin is taken up by passively by hepatocytes in the sinusoids and transported to the smooth endoplasmic reticulum by a protein called ligandin or Z protein. In the smooth endoplasmic reticulum bilirubin is conjugated to form water soluble bilirubin diglucuronide by UDP glucuronyltransferase. The activity of this enzyme can be induced by phenobarbitone.

Table 20.1. Summary of Haem metabolism

Product	Haem ▷ Biliverdin ▷ Unconjugated bilirubin ▷Conjugated bilirubin ▷Urobilinogen ▷Stercobilin
Location	Reticuloendothelial system Blood ▷ Liver ▷ Bile ducts ▷ Gall bladder ▷ Gut ▷ Gut bacteria
Colour	Red ▷ Green ▷Yellow ▷ Green/brown ▷ Colourless ▷ Brown
Enzyme	Haem oxygenase ▷Biliverdin reductase ▷UDP glucoronyltransferase

Conjugated bilirubin is actively transported into the bile ducts. The process of conjugation makes bilirubin water soluble and this easier to excrete. Once in the gut conjugated bilirubin is either hydrolyzed and reduced by bacteria in the gut to form urobilinogen a colourless compound or oxidized back to biliverdin giving bile its characteristic dark green colour. Most of the urobilinogen is eventually oxidized by intestinal bacteria to stercobilin, which gives stool its characteristic brown colour. Some of the urobilinogen is reabsorbed from the colon and enters the portal blood and the enterohepatic urobilinogen cycle in which it is taken up by the liver and then re-secreted into the bile. This process occurs more efficiently in the presence of increased bile acids. Bile acid malabsorption from any cause results in compensatory excretion of higher concentrations of bile salts which increases the risk of gallstones. The remainder of the urobilinogen is transported by the blood to the kidney. Here it is converted to yellow/orange urobilin and excreted.

Conjugated hyperbilirubinaemia (> 17 μmol/L if the total bilirubin is < 85 μmol/L or >20% of the total bilirubin) indicates cholestasis. Cholestasis may be a manifestation of generalized hepatocellular injury, obstruction to bile flow at any level of the biliary tree, or it may be caused by a specific problem with bile transport into the canaliculus. Pale stools in the presence of jaundice represent significant cholestasis due to obstruction of the bile flow.

Table 20.2 Differential Diagnosis of Neonatal Cholestasis (CAMOFLAGED)

Group of disorders	Examples
Congenital infection	TORCH, Syphilis, HIV
Acquired infection	Urinary tract infection, Sepsis
Metabolic	Galactosemia, Tyrosinemia, Defects in bile acid synthesis
Obstructive	Biliary atresia, choledochal cyst, inspissated bile syndrome
Flow (cholestasis)	Alagille syndrome, CF, progressive familial intrahepatic cholestasis
Alpha-1 antitrypsin	Alpha-1 antitrypsin deficiency
Generalised	Prematurity, cystic fibrosis, generalised illness, shock, heart failure
Endocrinopathy	Hypothyroidism, hypopituitarism
Drug or toxin	Parenteral nutrition

Biliary atresia (BA) is the commonest cause of neonatal cholestasis accounting for about 40-50% cases. BA is an evolving disease with inflammation and gradual destruction of the biliary ducts. The ducts are eventually replaced by scar tissue. Infants with BA typically are asymptomatic at birth and develop jaundice in the first few weeks after birth. Initially they feed well and thrive. As the bile flow diminishes, the stool colour loses its normal pigmentation and becomes acholic, or clay-coloured. The finding of pale stools in a jaundiced newborn should prompt investigations for BA. While biochemical tests confirm conjugated hyperbilirubinaemia and assess the liver function imaging studies such as ultra sound and HIDA (Hepatobiliary IminoDiacetic Acid) scans are used to identify the anatomical abnormality. Ultrasound may demonstrate absence of the gallbladder and no dilatation of the biliary tree but its main use is to rule out other anatomic abnormalities of the common bile duct, such as choledochal cysts. HIDA scans are more specific and assess the patency of the extrahepatic biliary system. Evidence of intestinal excretion of isotope confirms patency of the extrahepatic biliary system.

Breast milk Jaundice

This is a benign unconjugated hyperbilirubinaemia associated with breast feeding. It is a common cause of prolonged jaundice in the otherwise healthy breastfed infant born at term. Exact aetiology of this condition remains uncertain. Betaglucuronidase in breast milk is thought to play a part by causing deconjugation of bilirubin glucuronide in the gut and increasing enterohepatic circulation. Discontinuation of breast feeding leads to a rapid fall in bilirubin. There are no signs of dehydration or sepsis in our clinical case and whilst possible Hepatitis A is unlikely without a contact history. Liver function tests would reveal significant elevation of transaminases in children with hepatitis.

Syllabus Mapping

Gastroenterology and Hepatology

*   understand the role of the gut in homeostasis and its dysfunction
*   know the genetic and environmental factors in the aetiology of gut and liver disease

Neonatology

*   understand the physiology and principles of treatment of jaundice in the neonatal period

References

1. Brumbaugh D, Mack C. Conjugated hyperbilirubinemia in children. *Pediatr Rev* 2012;**33**:291-302.

2. Frederick J. Suchy, Ronald J. Sokol, William F. Balistreri. Liver Disease in children 3rd edition 2007; pp28-33.

3. Fischer JE, et al. Mastery of surgery: 5th (fifth) edition. 2006; Volume 1 pp 1188-1192.

Chapter 21: A teenager with an imprinting disorder Dr Natalie Smith

A 16 year old girl with known Prader-Willi syndrome secondary to uniparental disomy attends clinic with her parents. During discussion her parents ask you if she were to become pregnant whether the baby is likely to be born with Prader–Willi syndrome.

Q1. **What do you advise them about the recurrence risk?**

A. It depends on the sex of the baby
B. The baby has a 50% chance of having Angelman syndrome
C. The baby has a 50% chance of having PWS
D. You would expect the baby to be affected
E. You would expect the baby to be unaffected

Following the consultation you consider whether your advice would have been different if the Prader-Willi syndrome was the result of a chromosomal deletion.

Q2. **If the 16 year old child had Prader-Willi syndrome as a result of a chromosomal deletion what would be the recurrence risk of a related genetic disorder?**

A. It depends on the sex of the baby
B. The baby has a 50% chance of having Angelman syndrome
C. The baby has a 50% chance of having PWS
D. You would expect the baby to be affected
E. You would expect the baby to be unaffected

Answers and Rationale

Q1. **E. You would expect the baby to be unaffected**

Q2. **B. The baby would have a 50% chance of having Angelman syndrome**

Prader-Willi Syndrome (PWS) is a rare condition affecting less than 1 in 15,000 children born in the UK. It affects boys and girls equally and children of all ethnic backgrounds. Symptoms vary with age presenting with hypotonia in infancy followed by excessive eating, development of obesity and developmental delay in later childhood. Obstructive sleep apnoea syndrome is common as are hypogonadism and infertility. Angelman Syndrome (AS) is even rarer affecting about 1 in 25,000 people. This frequently presents with severe developmental delay evident by 6 – 12 months, ataxia, microcephaly and recurrent seizures. There are several characteristic behavioural signs including frequent smiling and laughter, excitability and hand flapping, a fascination with water and sleep difficulties which may be profound. Whilst the two conditions have profoundly different clinical features they are caused by deletion or loss of function of an identical part of the human genome. They are both the result of genomic imprinting. This question tests the candidates understanding of imprinting.

Imprinting

Genomic imprinting is a phenomenon that describes how the phenotypic expression of a gene depends on the parent of origin. It is generally accepted that each copy of an autosomal chromosome is functionally equivalent but this is not the case for all chromosomes or gene loci. In some cases the gene that is expressed depends on whether it has been inherited from the mother or from the father.

Prader-Willi and Angelman syndromes are examples of imprinting disorders caused by deletion of the same region on the long arm of chromosome 15 (15q11-13). This region of the human genome is host to a number of genes which are subject to genomic imprinting. Genes in this region are differentially silenced depending upon whether they are inherited from the mother or father of the child. Thus deletions of maternal or paternal genetic material lead to very different conditions in the progeny.

Deletion of this region (15 q11-13) of the paternal chromosome leads to loss of expression of up to seven genes which are jointly responsible for the expression of PWS. Whilst the child will inherit copies of these genes from their mother, they have been rendered functionally incompetent during oogenesis and function cannot be restored. Uniparental disomy (in the case of the 16 year old girl) describes that situation where both chromosomes from the pair have been inherited from one parent, in her case her mother. She does not carry a paternally derived chromosome 15 and therefore has inherited two sets of functionally incompetent genes. It is believed that the most common reason for this to occur is if the pregnancy starts off with a trisomy 15 and in order to survive the cell line must become disomic (as most trisomies are lethal). The random loss of one chromosome may lead to inheritance of two chromosomes from one parent. It is thought that about 30 % of cases of PWS are secondary to UPD.

Deletion of the maternal portion of this region of chromosome leads to AS. In a similar way UPD from the father leads to AS.

When the paternal gene is absent there is no expression of the genes in that region at all, since the corresponding maternal genes are usually silenced. The exact function of the genes involved has yet to be fully understood and so it is not clear why those with PWS display certain phenotypes. There has been no single gene mutation identified as a cause of PWS.

There has been a gene identified as responsible for Angelman syndrome – UBE3A. This is normally silenced on the paternal chromosome and the maternal copy is responsible for action in the brain. If the maternal gene is missing there is an insufficient amount of UBE3A in the brain which leads to problems seen in Angelman syndrome.

Once the principles underpinning imprinting disorders are understood it is relatively simple to answer the hypothetical questions set by the parents. In a child with PWS secondary to uniparental disomy we know that the genome is intact. Therefore, the process of oogenesis should 'reset' the imprinting and therefore the risk of recurrence of PWS (or indeed AS) is very low. Therefore the chances of this lady having a baby with PWS is approximately the same as for the general population which is <1%.

This girl in question 2 has PWS caused by a deletion on chromosome 15. This chromosome is paternally derived material as we know that absence of paternal genes in this area leads to PWS. If she decides to have a baby in the future she has a 50% chance of passing on a 'normal' chromosome 15 and a 50% chance of passing on the chromosome 15 containing the deletion. However, in this situation the child will have inherited the abnormal copy of chromosome 15 from its mother. The answer is therefore D. The baby has a 50 % chance of having Angelman syndrome as the deletion will be in the maternally derived chromosome.

In reality not many individuals with PWS go on to have children themselves but there have been some rare exceptions in females with the condition.

Syllabus Mapping

Genetics and Dysmorphology

- understand the scientific basis of genetic disorders and inheritance
- be able to construct a family tree and interpret patterns of inheritance
- understand the basis of molecular genetics including fluorescent in-situ hybridisation (FISH), uniparental disomy (UPD) and epigenetics
- understand the chromosomal and molecular basis of genetic disorders
- know the basis of genetic screening and diagnosis, the conditions for which they are used and the ethical dilemmas they pose

References

1. Nelson Textbook of Pediatrics, 19th Edition (2011) Chapters 75 and 76. Kliegman RM, Stanton B, St. Geme J, *et al.*

2. Illustrated Textbook of Paediatrics, 3rd Edition (2011), Chapter 8. Lissauer T.

3. www.nhs.uk/conditions/prader-willi-syndrome

4. www.nhs.uk/conditions/Angelman-syndrome

5. Nafee TM, Farrell WE, Carroll WD *et al.* Epigenetic control of fetal gene expression. BJOG 2008; **115**:158-68.

Chapter 22: The child with oligohydramnios
Dr Caroline Johnson

Lucy, a 28 year old woman in her first pregnancy, attends her 20/40 scan with her husband. They are a little concerned that Lucy's abdomen is not as big as it should be but are mostly just keen to find out the baby's gender and are excited to be told that they are expecting a baby boy.

Lucy is fit and well, on no medications apart from "pregnancy vitamins". Her husband, who is not related to her except by marriage, is also well.

The 20 week scan shows oligohydramnios.

Q1.   Which of the following mechanisms is most likely to result in oligohydramnios in the second half of pregnancy?

A.   Antenatal seizure activity
B.   Decreased fetal movements
C.   Increased fetal swallowing movements
D.   Reduced bowel motility
E.   Renal tract obstruction

Q2.   The ultrasonographer tells you that there is hydronephrosis evident on the scans. What is the most likely diagnosis?

A.   Amniotic fluid leakage
B.   Autosomal recessive polycystic kidney disease
C.   Duodenal obstruction due to annular pancreas
D.   Posterior urethral valves
E.   Potters syndrome

Q3.   The baby is born alive at 34 weeks. The most significant medical problem initially is likely to be:

A.   Intra-uterine growth restriction
B.   Prematurity
C.   Pulmonary hypoplasia
D.   Renal failure
E.   Talipes with contractures

Answers and Rationale

Q1.   E. Renal tract obstruction

Q2.   D. Posterior urethral valves

Q3.   C. Pulmonary hypolasia

Amniotic fluid surrounds the fetus from very early in pregnancy. Initially it is derived from maternal plasma and acts as a buffer/additional extracellular compartment. When the baby has too little amniotic fluid this is known as oligohydramnios. Polyhydramnios describes an excess of amniotic fluid.

By 8 weeks gestation the fetal urethra is patent. At about the same time the fetus starts to swallow the amniotic fluid and the primitive fetal kidneys begin to excrete urine. However, in the early stages of pregnancy amniotic fluid volume is predominantly influenced by fetal size, as fluid initially passes freely across the permeable surface membranes of the fetus. Therefore, even significant functional problems with the kidneys and renal tract may not be apparent on early dating scans.

This changes after 19 weeks gestation as the skin keratinises and becomes impermeable. After this time the amniotic fluid volume is affected much more by the fetus' ability to swallow and to excrete urine. The volume increases rapidly to reach a maximum of around 800ml at 34 weeks before reducing again towards term. By the second half of pregnancy (from 20 weeks onwards) it is the balance between fetal 'urination' and fetal swallowing that determine the volume of amniotic fluid.

Amniotic fluid is important because it allows baby to move and breathe, cushions against sudden sharp movements, helps to maintain a constant temperature, and contains factors which help with normal growth and development, in particular development of the lungs and gut. It also contains antimicrobial peptides to help protect against infection (1).

The initial amniotic fluid volume is low, approximately 30 ml at 10 weeks, and it increases proportionally with increases in fetal size. Whilst fetal swallowing movements are important, and reduced fetal swallowing as a result of muscle weakness may result in polyhydramnios, it is rare for the converse to occur. If extra amniotic fluid is swallowed by the baby then under normal circumstances this would simply be excreted by the kidneys.

Hydronephrosis describes abnormal dilatation of the renal pelvis with or without dilation of the calyces. It can be detected antenatally by ultrasound from 12-14 weeks gestation and is found in 1% of pregnancies. Antenatal renal pelvic dilatation is classified into mild (5-10mm), moderate (10-15mm) and severe (>15mm). The majority (80%) resolve either before or after birth but some cases are associated with abnormalities including vesico-ureteric reflux and urinary tract obstruction (PUJ or VUJ).

Given the information supplied in the initial history (the parents are expecting a boy) and the presence of hydronephrosis we can determine that the most likely cause of oligohydramnios in this case is a form of renal tract obstruction which affects boys. Posterior urethral valves (PUV) is a condition affecting only boys in which there is a membranous partial obstruction of the posterior urethra. The incidence of PUV remains relatively constant, at 1 in 5,000 live male births. Affected boys do not tend to have any other system disorder aside from associated renal dysfunction; however, a higher incidence of cryptorchidism compared to the normal population has been noted. This can lead to vesico-ureteric reflux, hydronephrosis and renal failure. Severely affected baby boys can develop oligohydramnios and pulmonary hypoplasia in utero. Most are born well but require surgery to remove the obstruction and careful monitoring of any reflux/renal impairment. PUV and its consequences, including renal dysplasia, upper tract dilatation, vesico-ureteric reflux, urinary tract infection and bladder dysfunction, account for 25 – 30 % of paediatric renal transplantations in the UK (UK Transplant Registry) (2).

Potters syndrome is named after Emily Potter who described it in 1946 (3). She described infants with bilateral renal agenesis (no kidneys) and those problems resulting from it such as pulmonary hypoplasia and classic facial features including a beaked nose and low set ears. Potter sequence is where these features are present due to severe oligohydramnios of another cause.

Amniotic fluid leakage is another important cause of oligohydramnios. It is caused by rupture of the fetal membranes. This can occur at any point during the pregnancy. The membranes help to protect the baby from infection. Their rupture makes the baby vulnerable to infection, known as chorioamnionitis. The timing of the membrane rupture is important because risk of infection/preterm labour increases with duration of membrane rupture and pulmonary hypoplasia is more likely if oligohydramnios occurs before 26 weeks. Whilst aminiotic fluid leakage cannot be excluded in the case described it does not explain the observed hydronephrosis. Because of the risk of infection it should be considered in all cases of oligohydramnios.

Autosomal recessive polycystic kidney disease is a rare condition which leads to multiple cysts in both kidneys. The prognosis is relatively poor with a significant number of infants dying due to pulmonary hypoplasia and many others progressing rapidly to end stage renal failure.

Any form of bowel obstruction will potentially lead to polyhydramnios. Annular pancreas occurs in 1 in 12,000 live births and can cause obstruction by encircling the duodenum. When the fetus swallows amniotic fluid it is unable to pass through the gut and so there is an excess of amniotic fluid, known as polyhydramnios. Whilst annular pancreas is relatively common it often remains undiagnosed and roughly half of those with the condition do present with symptoms until adult life (4). Other causes of polyhydramnios include oesophageal atresia, any other cause of GI tract obstruction, maternal diabetes and neuromuscular conditions leading to poor fetal swallow.

For question 3, whilst all of the suggestions may be significant medical problems for the baby the most significant issue initially is pulmonary hypoplasia because where this is severe it may be incompatible with life/require ventilator support.

Syllabus Mapping

Genetics and dysmorphology

*   know the environmental factors which may affect prenatal development

Neonatology

*   understand the embryology of the human fetus from conception to birth and how errors in this process can lead to diseases or congenital anomalies
*   understand the normal physiological processes occurring during the perinatal period

Nephro-urology

*   understand the scientific basis of imaging and physiological investigations used in renal disorders
*   understand the disease associations of renal conditions with other conditions

References

1. Underwood MA, Gilbert WM, Sherman MP. Amniotic fluid: not just fetal urine anymore. *Journal of Perinatology* 2005;**25(5)**:341–348.

2. Steven LC, Desai D. Posterior urethral valves. Paediatric urology book, online at http://www. pediatricurologybook.com/urethral_valves.html [accessed 15th March 2013].

3. Potter EL. Facial characteristics in infants with bilateral renal agenesis. *Am J Obstet Gynecol* 1946;**51**:885.

4. Semrin MG, Russo MA. Anatomy, histology, embryology, and developmental anomalies of the stomach and duodenum. In: Feldman M, Friedman LS, Brandt LJ, eds. *Sleisenger & Fordtran's Gastrointestinal and Liver Disease*. 9th ed. Philadelphia, Pa: Saunders Elsevier; 2010: Chapter 45.

Chapter 23: The child with trisomy 21
Dr Caroline Johnson

Jennifer, a baby girl born to healthy unrelated parents, was reviewed at 36 hours of age because she was "floppy." On examination she is well but in addition to the hypotonia has Brushfield spots, single palmar creases and an increased sandal gap.

Q1.   Chromosomes are sent. If Jennifer does have Down's Syndrome the most likely result is:

A.   45 X0
B.   45,XX,der(14;21)(q10;q10)
C.   46,XY,+21
D.   47,XX,+18
E.   47,XX,+21

Q2.   In Down's syndrome the most likely cause of the additional chromosomal material is:

A.   Inherited translocation
B.   Maternal nondisjunction
C.   Mosaicism
D.   Paternal nondisjunction
E.   Spontaneous translocation

The family come back to see you. Both parents have been tested and shown to have normal chromosomes. The mother is now 35 years old.

Q3.   What is their risk of having another affected child?

A.   1%
B.   1% plus age adjusted risk
C.   2.5%
D.   25%
E.   25% plus age adjusted risk

Q4. Concerning screening: are the following statements are TRUE (T) or FALSE (F)?

A.   After 16 weeks screening is not helpful and parents should be offered diagnostic testing
B.   Amniocentesis can be performed in the first trimester
C.   Chorionic villus sampling can be performed from 10 weeks gestation
D.   The combined test will identify more than 90% of cases of T21
E.   The risk of miscarriage with amniocentesis and chorionic villus sampling is similar

Answers and Rationale

Q1.   **E. 47,XX,+21**
Q2.   **B. Maternal nondisjunction**
Q3.   **B. 1% plus age adjusted risk**
Q4.   **A. False B. False C. True D. False E. True**

Creation of a new baby begins at fertilisation when sperm from the male fuses with the egg from the female to make a zygote. But before fertilization occurs both the male and female germ cells undergo meiosis, the process in which the number of chromosomes in each cell is reduced from 46 (diploid) to 23 (haploid). Meiosis occurs in two stages; the first and second meiotic divisions.

Just prior to the first division each cell replicates its DNA leading to 46 "double chromosomes." These chromosomes then pair up with the other similar chromosomes – e.g. both Chromosome 21's. There is then a line formed between the pair, known as chiasma formation. This process allows the exchange of information, producing genetic variability. The pairs then pull apart and move to opposite ends of the cell in preparation for the cell dividing. Each cell then contains 23 "double chromosomes" and therefore the same genetic information as a somatic cell. The second meiotic division then occurs in which each of the double chromosomes split with each half moving to opposite ends of the cell which then divides to leave each germ cell with 23 chromosomes; 22 somatic and 1 sex chromosome.

Nondisjunction occurs when, during the first meiotic division a paired chromosome fails to separate, so that when cell division occurs one cell has two copies and one no copy of that chromosome. When fertilization subsequently occurs the resulting individual has three copies of that chromosome, known as a trisomy. Trisomy of chromosome 21 is known as Down's syndrome. The two other most common trisomies are trisomy 18 (Edward's Syndrome) and trisomy 13 (Patau's Syndrome). The process of nondisjunction can occur in either the maternal or paternal germ cells. Trisomy 21 occurs due to maternal nondisjunction in 88% of cases and paternal nondisjunction in 8%. In contrast to other trisomies it is survivable because of the relatively smaller number of genes present on chromosome 21 (there is a low gene density on a small chromosome).

Mosaicism occurs when nondisjunction occurs during a mitotic division in the embryotic cell (mitotic nondisjunction). This leads to an individual in which some cells have normal chromosomes and other cells have an abnormal amount of genetic material. The clinical features depend on which chromosome is affected and the percentage and distribution of cells involved. Mosaicism accounts for 1-2% of cases of Trisomy 21.

Translocation. When, during the process of meiosis, chromosomes pair and separate breaks can occur. The "broken" fragment of a chromosome can then become attached to another chromosome. This is known as a translocation. An example is where material from chromosome 21 is translocated onto chromosome 14. In some cases a translocation and subsequent cell division leads to a cell with the correct amount of genetic material – a so-called balanced translocation. Where genetic material is gained or lost as a result of the translocation and subsequent cell division the embryo created may have a lethal abnormality/genetic syndrome. Individuals who carry a balanced translocation will be normal but have an increased risk of having offspring with an unbalanced translocation.

Downs' Syndrome

Downs' Syndrome was first described by Langdon Down in 1866. Incidence increases with maternal age. Characteristic features include; microcephaly, brachycephaly, upslanting palpebral fissures, wide flat nasal bridge, Brushfield spots (white spots in the irises), 5th finger clinodactyly, single transverse palmar creases and an increased sandal gap (space between first and second toes). Children with Downs' Syndrome are generally hypotonic. They have learning difficulties and reach milestones such as walking later than other children. 40% of children with trisomy 21 have congenital heart disease. The most common cardiac malformations are atrio-venticular septal defect (AVSD), ventriculoseptal defect (VSD) and Fallot's tetralogy. Babies with Down's syndrome are also more likely to be born with duodenal atresia and to develop leukaemia or Alzheimer's disease as they get older.

Women in the UK are offered screening for Trisomy 21 at several stages of pregnancy.

The Combined Test consists of an ultrasound and a blood test. The ultrasound, between 11+2/40 and 14+1/40 weeks gestation measures the baby to estimate gestation and also the nuchal fold. The blood tests measures PAPP-A (pregnancy associated plasma protein-A) and free B-hCG (B-human chorionic gonadotrophin). The USS and blood results are combined with maternal age to give an estimated risk of Downs' syndrome in the fetus. The combined test picks up 84% of babies with Downs' Syndrome. There is a 2.2% false positive rate.

Quadruple test. Women who present/decide too late in pregnancy to have the combined test may have the quadruple test – a blood test which measures AFP, beta HCG, inhibin-A and oestriol and uses the results in combination with maternal age and gestation to calculate a risk of Downs' syndrome or spina bifida.

Women whose risk of Downs' Syndrome is greater than 1 in 150 are offered a diagnostic test to see if the baby is affected. A low risk result does not mean the baby does not have Downs' syndrome. Diagnostic tests are chorionic villus sampling (CVS) and amniocentesis:

CVS – This can be performed from 10-13 weeks gestation. A small needle is passed through the abdomen to remove cells from the placenta for chromosomal analysis. There is a 1% risk of miscarriage.

Amniocentesis – A needle is used to remove a sample of the amniotic fluid from the womb, usually between 16-20 weeks gestation but it can be done later. Cells from the fluid are then analysed. The miscarriage risk is quoted as 1%.

20 week anomaly scan – This scan looks at the developing fetus in detail system by system and can pick up both chromosomal and structural abnormalities.

Syllabus Mapping

Genetics and dysmorphology

The candidate must:

- understand the scientific basis of genetic disorders and inheritance
- understand the chromosomal and molecular basis of genetic disorders
- know the basis of genetic screening and diagnosis, the conditions for which they are used and the ethical dilemmas they pose

References and Further Reading

1. Patton MA. Chapter 12. Genetics. Forfar and Arneils Textbook of Paediatrics. Sixth Edition. Churchill Livingstone 2003.

2. Langmans Medical Embryology. Seventh Edition. TW Sadler 1995.

3. www.nhs.uk. http://www.nhs.uk/conditions/pregnancy-and-baby/pages/screening-amniocentesis-downs-syndrome.aspx#close (accessed 20th August 2013).

Chapter 24: Recurrence risk in conditions with known inheritance Dr Sam Behjati

You see a 9 month old girl of African descent who has been referred to you because of painful finger swelling. You diagnose dactylitis and suspect underlying sickle cell disease, which is confirmed by electrophoresis. Her mother, Brenda, has always been well. You have an electrophoresis result of the girl's father, Adam, on the hospital's computer system that tells you that he is not a carrier. Adam tells you that Brenda has recently fallen pregnant again.

Q1. **What is the probability that Adam and Brenda's unborn child will have sickle cell disease?**

A. 0%

B. 25%

C. 33%

D. 50%

E. It cannot be predicted as in sickle cell disease there is no correlation between genotype and phenotype

Q2. **A man has an X-linked monogenetic disease with complete penetrance. Looking at the family tree below, what is the risk of his daughter having his disease?**

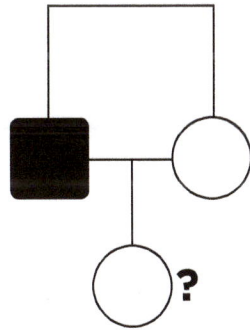

A. 50% if it is a dominant gene defect

B. 100% if it is a dominant gene defect

C. 75% if it is a dominant gene defect

D. 0% if it is a recessive gene defect

E. 50% if it is a recessive gene defect

Answers and Rationale

Q1.   **A. 0%**
Q2.   **B. 100% if it is a dominant gene defect**

Paediatric exams and general paediatric practice require a working knowledge of inheritance patterns of genetic diseases. When a disease is caused by mutations in a single gene (monogenic conditions), it is usually straightforward to answer questions about the recurrence risk of the disease. The picture gets more complicated if: diseases are caused by mutations in multiple genes; the mutation is present in some but not all tissues (mosaicism); there is no predictable correlation between the presence of a mutation and the clinical phenotype; gene function depends on whether the gene is maternally or paternally derived (imprinting); the affected gene is mitochondrial. The discussion below focuses on determining the recurrence risk of monogenic autosomal and X-linked diseases with known inheritance. Despite the apparent simplicity of this type of question, they are frequently answered incorrectly in the MRCPCH exam. Therefore a brief reminder of the basic principles is included here.

In order to determine the recurrence risk of genetic diseases with known inheritance, you need to know:

1) Is the mutation dominant or recessive?

2) Is the affected gene on a sex chromosome (X,Y) or on an autosome (chromosomes 1-22)?

3) Who in the family has the disease (the family tree)?

Each of those points is explained below.

1) Is the mutation dominant or recessive?

We have in our genomes two copies (alleles) of each gene, one inherited from each parent. One, or both of these genes, may harbour mutations. These mutations may render the gene malfunctional. When a single malfunctional gene suffices to cause disease, no matter how well the second copy of the gene functions, the genetic disease is referred to as being "dominant". When two defunct genes are required for a disease to occur, the disease is considered to be "recessive". As a rule of thumb (with many exceptions!), most diseases caused by gene defects in structural genes are dominant (e.g., osteogenesis imperfecta) whereas metabolic genetic diseases are recessive (e.g., phenolketonuria).

2) Is the affected gene on a sex chromosome (X,Y) or on an autosome (chromosomes 1-22)?

Carriers of mutated autosomal genes causing recessive disorders never develop the disease. This is not the case for recessive genes that are on sex chromosomes. Mutations in such genes may or may not cause disease in children of affected parents, depending on whether it is a boy or a girl who inherits the mutated gene. An example is glucose-6-phosphate (G6PD) deficiency, an X-linked recessive disorder. If a boy inherits a defunct copy of the G6PD gene, which lies on the X chromosome, he will get the disease. If a girl, however, inherits the defunct gene she will not get the disease (provided she inherited a functioning copy from the other parent). In X-linked dominant conditions (e.g. haemophilia A,B), however, girls will also get the disease if they inherit the mutated gene because the normal copy they have cannot compensate for the malfunctioning copy.

3) Who in the family has the disease (the family tree)?

You need this information to determine the risk of a mutated gene being passed on. You can also use family trees to determine the mode of inheritance of a genetic disease that is present in a family and this is a particularly common type of question in the MRCPCH Theory and Science exam.

Using these three pieces of information, we can now turn back to the questions.

Question 1

Sickle cell disease is a monogenetic, autosomal recessive condition with complete penetrance. Disease severity is variable but whether or not someone has the disease can always be predicted from their genotype. If the child does have Sickle cell disease, she must have inherited two mutated copies of the haemoglobin gene. The proposed father has two normal copies of the gene. Therefore, it is likely that the proposed father is not the biological father of the child. Non-paternity is common and occurs in 10-15% of the UK population. The mother is either a carrier or unaffected as she has always been well. In either case the correct answer is A, 0%. A mother who is a carrier and a father who has two normal genes will together never have a child with Sickle cell disease. An alternative, exceedingly unlikely explanation is that in addition to the mutation she inherited from her mother, the girl developed a de novo mutation in the other copy of the gene.

Question 2

As a man, the father only has a single copy of the X-chromosome and therefore carries one copy of the mutated gene and no other copy of the gene. His wife carries two normal copies of the gene. Each parent passes on a single sex chromosome to their progeny. Mothers always supply an X chromosome. Therefore the sex of the offspring will tell us which sex chromosome father supplied. Sons always receive a Y chromosome from their father and daughters always receive the X chromosome. Their daughter will therefore always inherit a mutated copy of the gene (from the father). If the gene defect is dominant, her chances of having the disease would therefore be 100%. If the gene defect is recessive, she will not have the disease.

Syllabus Mapping

Although we chose to construct a question on sickle cell disease it is worth noting that for most systems the new syllabus recommends that there is an understanding of the genetic factors which underpin disorders.

Our questions map to:

Haematology and oncology

•   know the genetic and environmental factors in the aetiology of haematological disorders and malignancies

Genetics and dysmoprhology

•   understand the scientific basis of genetic disorders and inheritance
•   be able to construct a family tree and interpret patterns of inheritance
•   understand the chromosomal and molecular basis of genetic disorders

References

1.   Helen M. Kingston. ABC of Clinical Genetics. 3rd edition. Wiley-Blackwell; 2002.

Chapter 25: The child with severe anaemia
Dr Jill Mant, Dr Vasanta Nanduri

A 4 year old Caucasian girl presents to the emergency department with a short history of fever and lethargy. On examination she looks extremely pale and has moderate splenomegaly. Her mum reports that she is normally an active girl but has been tired recently.

She developed jaundice requiring phototherapy soon after birth and since then she has had intermittent episodes of jaundice. Her father had a cholecystectomy at the age of 25.

Initial blood results show:

Hb 2.8 g/dL
WBC 5.3 x10⁹/L
Neutrophils 3.2 x10⁹/L
Platelets 180 x10⁹/L
Reticulocytes 0.1%

Questions

Q1. Choose the ONE most likely diagnosis:

A.   Acute lymphoblastic leukaemia
B.   Aplastic anaemia secondary to Hepatitis B infection
C.   Glucose-6-phosphate dehydrogenase (G6PD) deficiency with an acute haemolytic crisis
D.   Hereditary spherocytosis with an acute aplastic crisis
E.   Sickle cell anaemia with an acute aplastic crisis

Q2. Choose the ONE most appropriate next treatment step:

A.   Antithymocyte globulin (ATG)
B.   Blood transfusion
C.   Erythropoietin
D.   Intravenous immunoglobulin
E.   Splenectomy

Answers and Rationale

Q1. **D. Hereditary spherocytosis with an acute aplastic crisis**
Q2. **B. Blood transfusion**

In the human fetus clusters of stem cells (called blood islands) are first seen in the yolk sac during the 3rd week of embryonic development. By about 3 months of development these cells migrate to the liver which becomes the main site of blood production. The bone marrow gradually takes over synthesis from about 5 months and by birth almost all red cells are made in the bone marrow. In children the entire skeleton is haematopoietically active. Bone marrow contains pluripotent haematopoietic stem cells that proliferate and differentiate to form the different elements of blood including erythrocytes. Once mature, the erythrocytes are released into the systemic circulation. Immature red cells are called reticulocytes and usually comprise about 1% of circulating red cells. A normal red blood cell has a life span of 120 days after which it is destroyed by the phagocytic cells of the spleen. Erythropoiesis is regulated by the hormone erythropoietin (EPO) which is synthesised predominantly in the kidney (90%) and to a lesser extent by the liver (10%).

Anaemia can be caused by inadequate red cell production, loss of red cells or premature destruction of red cells. It is usually possible to differentiate between the above causes by looking at the patient's red cell indices, reticulocyte count, blood film and bilirubin. The main causes are summarised below (Table 25.1).

Table 25.1 Causes of anaemia in childhood

Cause of anaemia	Clinical examples
Inadequate production	Bone Marrow Failure e.g. Aplastic anaemia, virus infection Haematinic deficiency e.g. Iron deficiency Decreased erythropoietin drive e.g. Chronic renal failure Ineffective erythropoiesis e.g. β–Thalassaemia
Red cell loss	Acute blood loss e.g. Trauma Occult / chronic blood loss e.g. GI bleeding from Crohn's disease, menorrhagia
Premature red cell destruction (haemolysis)	Red cell membrane defects e.g. Hereditary Spherocytosis Red cell enzyme defects e.g. G6PD deficiency Haemoglobin defects e.g. Sickle cell disease and thalassaemia Immune mediated red cell destruction e.g. alloimmune – Haemolytic disease of the newborn, or autoimmune – secondary to EBV or mycoplasma Non-immune mediated acquired red cell destruction e.g. Haemolytic uraemic syndrome, malaria, septicaemia

Bone marrow failure is associated with a low reticulocyte count. It can be caused by marrow infiltration (e.g. acute lymphoblastic leukaemia or neuroblastoma) or aplastic anaemia. Aplastic anaemia is characterised by marrow hypoplasia and a peripheral pancytopenia (low haemoglobin, white cell count and platelets). The pluripotent stem cells are affected with reduction in all cell lines. The cause of aplastic anaemia is often unknown. About 20% are inherited, with Fanconi anaemia being the most common inherited aplastic anaemia. Of the acquired forms, many are idiopathic. Recognised triggers include viral infections (CMV, Non-A, non-B hepatitis, HIV, EBV), drugs (acetazolamide, chloramphenicol, chemotherapy) and whole body irradiation. Aplastic anaemia is initially managed with supportive treatment with blood and platelet transfusions and treatment of infections. If an HLA-matched donor is available, bone marrow transplant is often the treatment of choice. If a suitable donor is not available, immune suppression with antithymocyte globulin (ATG) and cyclosporin can be used.

Parvovirus B19 can cause bone marrow failure but it usually selectively replicates in the erythroid progenitor cells resulting in isolated red cell aplasia. In most patients this is sub-clinical but in patients with an underlying chronic haemolytic disorder and reduced red cell lifespan (e.g. hereditary spherocytosis or sickle cell anaemia) it can result in severe life threatening aplastic anaemia. The infection is typically self-limiting and lasts 10-14 days. During this time patients may require multiple blood transfusions. Parvovirus can also cause a more chronic infection in immunocompromised patients.

Premature red cell destruction is usually associated with a high reticulocyte count. There is an accumulation of products of haemoglobin catabolism (resulting in a high unconjugated bilirubin) and a marked increase in erythropoiesis within the bone marrow to compensate for red cell loss. Clinically patients may have jaundice (including neonatal jaundice), gallstones and splenomegaly. Haemolytic anaemia can be inherited or acquired. Inherited disorders include red cell membrane defects, red cell enzyme defects and haemoglobin defects.

Hereditary spherocytosis is the most common hereditary haemolytic anaemia in northern Europeans. Most cases show autosomal dominant inheritance although there is a more severe autosomal recessive variant. The genetic abnormality results in defects in proteins of the red cell cytoskeleton. Spectrin defect is the most common abnormality but ankyrin, band 3 and band 4.2 defects are also known. The membrane defects result in the erythrocytes being spheroidal, less deformable, and vulnerable to splenic sequestration and destruction. On average they have a life span of only 28 days. Haemolysis leads to jaundice and gallstone formation. The severity of the disease can vary and is often classified as mild, moderate or severe based on the haemoglobin, bilirubin, reticulocyte count and the erythrocytic spectrin concentration. Treatment depends on severity. All patients with moderate and severe disease should receive daily folic acid to support the increase in erythropoeisis. There is debate about whether patients with mild disease also need folic acid. Splenectomy is the treatment of choice for severe disease and for many patients with moderate disease. Splenectomy reduces haemolysis leading to a significant prolongation of red cell lifespan. However, splenectomy is associated with an increased risk of life threatening sepsis from encapsulated organisms (especially S pneumoniae). If possible splenectomy should be delayed until the patient is at least 6 years old and all patients should be vaccinated against pneumococcus, Haemophilus, meningococcus and Hepatitis B as well as treated with lifelong penicillin prophylaxis (1,2).

In the above case, the history of jaundice suggests a possible haemolytic disorder. There was also a family history of gallstones which could suggest a family history of chronic haemolysis. This would be in keeping with hereditary spherocytosis, G6PD deficiency or sickle cell anaemia. The fact that the patient is a girl (G6PD deficiency is normally X-linked) and Caucasian (sickle cell disease is very rare in Caucasians) makes hereditary spherocytosis the most likely diagnosis. At the time of the acute presentation the patient is very anaemic with a low reticulocyte count which suggests decreased production and not acute haemolysis. The child is most likely suffering an acute aplastic crisis secondary to parvovirus infection. If the child had acute lymphoblastic leukaemia or aplastic anaemia due to hepatitis, one would expect all of the cell lines to be affected and not just the haemoglobin. The answer to question 1 is therefore D. Hereditary spherocytosis with an acute aplastic crisis.

An aplastic crisis due to parvovirus is normally self limiting in children with hereditary spherocytosis and treatment is supportive with blood transfusions as necessary (1,2) [Answer B. Blood transfusion]. The child may benefit from a splenectomy in the future but ideally this would be delayed until she was over 6 years old and otherwise well. Erythropoietin levels are high in children with hereditary spherocytosis and it has no role in this girl's treatment. Erythropoietin is frequently used in children with chronic renal failure who have reduced erythropoietin levels and associated anaemia. Antithymocyte globulin (ATG) is immunosuppressive but is unlikely to help as the underlying problem here is not autoimmune. Similarly, intravenous immunoglobulin is not likely to help although it has been used in children with immunodeficiencies and chronic parvovirus infection (3).

Syllabus Mapping

Haematology and oncology

- understand the changes in haematopoiesis that occur throughout childhood
- know the genetic and environmental factors in the aetiology of haematological disorders and malignancies
- understand the physiological basis of haematopoiesis and how diseases including infections, impact upon this
- understand the pathophysiology of disorders of haematopoiesis, coagulation and malignancy
- understand the basis of treatment for anaemias, disorders of coagulation and malignancies

References

1. Bolton-Maggs PHB, *et al.* Guidelines for the diagnosis and management of hereditary spherocytosis – 2011 update. *Br J Haematol* 2012;**156**:37–49.

2. Bolton-Maggs PHB, *et al.* Guidelines for the diagnosis and management of hereditary spherocytosis. *Br J Haematol* 2004;**126**:455–474.

3. Crabol Y, *et al.* Intravenous immunoglobulin therapy for pure red cell aplasia related to human parvovirus B19 infection: a retrospective study of 10 patients and a review of the literature. *Clin Infect Dis* 2013;**56(7)**:968-77.

Chapter 26: A child with pain in her hands and feet Dr Will Carroll, Lisa Carroll

A 6 year old girl with known sickle cell disease is admitted to the children's ward with pain in the hands and feet. She has been started on intravenous fluids and given oral morphine and oxygen. You are called to review her on the ward.

Q1. **Which ONE of the following complications of sickle cell disease is more common in early childhood compared to the older population?**

A.   Bacterial infection
B.   Chest crisis
C.   Gallstones
D.   Osteonecrosis
E.   Painful crisis

Q2. **What treatment will be most likely to immediately improve her pain control?**

A.   Broad spectrum antibiotics
B.   Dexamethasone
C.   Folic acid
D.   Hydroxycarbamide (hydroxyurea)
E.   Intravenous (parenteral) opiates

Q3 **Which ONE of the following factors is best associated with increased risk of painful crises during childhood?**

A.   Thalassaemia trait
B.   Lower fetal haemoglobin concentration
C.   Lower granulocyte (neutrophil) count
D.   Lower haematocrit
E.   Younger age

Answers and Rationale

Q1. **Bacterial infection**

Q2. **Dexamethasone**

Q3. **Lower fetal haemoglobin concentration**

Sickle cell disease is one of the commonest single gene diseases in the world. It is caused by a single mutation in the β-globin gene that results in a substitution of a valine for glutamic acid. Despite the apparent genetic simplicity there are considerable variation in clinical severity and the pattern of expression seen between individuals and in the same individual over a lifetime. These differences are believed to relate to differences in the overall concentration of sickle cell haemoglobin within red cells of affected individuals. The two best established genetic modifiers are determinants of fetal haemoglobin concentrations and co-inheritance of α-thalassemia (1).

Adult-type haemoglobin is usually made up of two β-globin and two β-globin chains. The substitution of valine for glutamic acid at the sixth amino acid in the β-globin chain changes the biophysical properties of the adult-type haemoglobin chains so that they are predisposed to polymerise following deoxygenation (2). In those with sickle cell disease the adult haemoglobin has two abnormal β-globin molecules and is denoted HbS. Once more than half of the circulating haemoglobin is HbS then individuals will express the disease, thus individuals with one defective β-globin gene will be asymptomatic. The rate and extent of HbS polymerisation is proportional to the extent and duration of haemoglobin deoxygenation, the intracellular HbS concentration (to about the 34th power) and the presence of fetal haemoglobin in the erythrocyte, which effectively reduces the concentration of HbS. Polymerisation leads to erythrocyte rigidity and characteristic changes in their shape to form pointed sickle cells.

The maintenance of high fetal haemoglobin concentrations beyond infancy ameliorates most aspects of sickle cell disease. The relatively higher concentrations of fetal haemoglobin in younger children reduces the risk of most sickle cell complications with the exception of bacterial infection which are a major cause of morbidity and mortality in children with sickle-cell disease. The increased susceptibility to infection is probably multifactorial with impaired splenic function and defects in complement activation being commonly seen. Several organisms including S pneumoniae, H influenza, and Salmonella species are important infections and children benefit from both penicillin prophylaxis and immunisation with conjugate vaccines against S pneumoniae and H influenza type b.

α-thalassaemia trait exists in almost a third of children of African origin with sickle-cell disease and more than half of those from India and Saudi Arabia. α-thalassaemia reduces the concentration of haemoglobin in each erythrocyte, decreasing the tendency of HbS to polymerise which results in increased haemoglobin concentrations and decreased rates of haemolysis. The clinical effects of α-thalassaemia are variable but generally variable decreasing the risk of stroke, gall stones, leg ulcers and priapism but the frequency of painful crises is not reduced (3). Of the laboratory variables which can be measured only haematocrit and fetal haemoglobin concentration are associated with the rate of painful crises (3). Children with a higher haematocrit or lower fetal haemoglobin are at increased risk of painful crises.

Treatments for sickle cell disease rely on the known physiology. Therefore acute painful crises are treated with supplemental oxygen, intravenous fluids and pain relief. Acute pain is the most common reason for admission to hospital for all age groups but it is more common in teenagers and adults than younger children. Opiate analgesia is effective but oral opiates appear to be as effective as parenteral opiates in children (4). The UK confidential enquiry into deaths of patients with sickle-cell disease identified opiate-related oversedation as an important cause of death (5). Corticosteroids are known to be effective in shortening episodes of acute pain, although the use of steroids has mostly stopped because of a high frequency of rebound pain and hospital re-admission. Whilst antibiotics, folic acid and hydroxycarbamide are all used in children with sickle cell disease to prevent complications but are not effective acutely.

Acute chest syndrome is the second commonest cause of hospitalisation in children with sickle-cell disease. It results from a combination of infection, fat embolism and vaso-occlusion of the pulmonary vessels. It is a serious complication with a significant minority (13%) requiring mechanical ventilation and a 3% mortality rate. Chest X-ray demonstrates the presence of new pulmonary y infiltrates. Treatment involves broad-spectrum antibiotics, bronchodilators and oxygen. Blood transfusion can be useful if the haemoglobin has fallen dramatically and dexamethasone is known to reduce the need for this.

Crises can be prevented by increasing the fetal haemoglobin concentrations. Many cytotoxic drugs increase fetal haemoglobin concentrations. Hydroxycarbamide (hydroxyurea) was initially used in sickle cell disease because it is effective orally and has low toxic effects (6) but it has other potentially beneficial effects including reduced platelet and white cell counts and increased nitric oxide production. Hydroxycarbamide should be considered for children with recurrent episodes of acute pain (more than 3 per year) or for those with more than one episode of acute sickle chest syndrome in 2 years (7). In general it is well tolerated with its main side-effect being a dose-dependent myelosuppression. In most forms of sickle-cell disease there is an accompanying haemolytic anaemia which may increase folate requirements and hence folate supplementation is often necessary.

Blood transfusion has an established role in the management of acute and chronic complications in sickle-cell disease. Transfusion corrects anaemia whilst reducing the percentage of HbS, suppresses HbS synthesis and reduces haemolysis. However, repeated blood transfusion is inevitably associated with iron overload. Therefore, iron chelation therapy is important in those requiring regular transfusions. Stroke is relatively common and occurs in about 1 in 10 children with sickle-cell disease. The risk of stroke appears to be significantly reduced in children receiving regular transfusions when compared to therapy with hydroxycarbamide (8).

Syllabus Mapping

Haematology and oncology

The candidate must:

- understand the changes in haematopoiesis that occur throughout childhood
- know the genetic and environmental factors in the aetiology of haematological disorders and malignancies
- understand the pathophysiology of disorders of haematopoiesis
- understand the basis of treatment for anaemias

References

1. Rees DC, William TN, Gladwin MT. Sickle-cell disease. *Lancet* 2010;**376**:2018-31.

2. Steinberg MH. Management of sickle cell disease *New Engl J Med* 1999;**340**:1021-1030.

3. Platt OS, et al. Pain in sickle cell disease. Rates and risk factors. *N Engl J Med* 1991;**325**:11-6.

4. Jacobson SJ, Kopecky BA, Joshi P, Babul N. Randomized trial of oral morphine for painful episodes of sickle-cell disease in children. *Lancet* 1997;**350**:1358-61.

5. National Confidential Enquiry into Patient Outcome and Death. A sickle crisis? A report of the National Confidential Enquiry Into Patient Outcome and Death (2008). http://www.ncepod.org.uk/2008report1/Downloads/Sickle_report.pdf

6. Platt OS, Orkin SH, Dover G, Beardsley GP, Miller B, Nathan DG. Hydroxyurea enhances fetal hemoglobin production in sickle cell anaemia. *J Clin Invest* 1984;**74**:652-56.

7. BNF for children July 2013-2014. p452.

8. Ware RE et al. Stroke With Transfusions Changing to Hydroxyurea (SWiTCH). *Blood* 2012;**119**:3925-32.

Chapter 27: The child with unexplained bruising Dr Karen Aucott

The following are causes of bruising in childhood:

A. A deficiency of factor VIII
B. Decreased production of intrinsically defective platelets
C. Drug induced thrombocytopenia
D. IgA immune complex deposition in small vessels
E. Inherited bleeding tendency caused by an abnormality on chromosome 12
F. Splenic destruction of antibody coated platelets
G. Toxin related endothelial injury, thrombus formation and platelet consumption
H. Trauma/Non accidental injury
I. Unregulated activation of the clotting pathway leading to excess fibrin clots

For each of the cases below, select one answer from the list which best describes the pathophysiological process for the most likely diagnosis.

Q1. A 6 year old girl presents to the emergency department with a widespread purpuric rash. She had been sent home from school that morning as she was feeling generally unwell. At bedtime her mother noticed a widespread rash which did not disappear on the glass test. On arrival, she was pyrexial, tachycardic and hypotensive.

Q2. A 4 year old boy is seen in CED as his parents noticed that he had multiple bruises over his limbs, trunk and back. He had had a sore throat a few weeks previously but is otherwise well and cheerfully playing. He has epilepsy which is well controlled with lamotrogine. Examination is unremarkable other than atopic eczema.

Q3. A 2 year old child is referred by the health visitor with a right periorbital bruise. Her mother does not know how it happened but an older sibling says that she fell off the top bunk. The child is quiet but aside from the bruise examination is unremarkable.

Q4. A 4 year old girl is admitted to hospital with a fever, bloody diarrhoea and vomiting. She initially improved with oral rehydration solution but later became irritable. Her parents feel she is not herself and are worried because she has a petechial rash and looks puffy.

Q5. Simon is 6 years old and presents to the emergency department with an urticarial rash to his lower limbs and some purpura. He has had some colicky abdominal pain but is otherwise well. Examination reveals mild swelling of the ankles bilaterally and an urticarial maculopapular rash to his legs and buttocks with some developing purpura.

Q6. A 7 year old child attends CED with a prolonged nosebleed and is also noted to have scattered bruises. His mother doesn't know how he got them but says that both him and his sister seem to get a bruise just by walking past furniture; she separated from their father before they were born but thinks that he may have bruised easily as well.

Answers and Rationale

Q1. **I. Unregulated activation of the clotting pathway leading to excess fibrin clots**

Q2. **F. Splenic destruction of antibody coated platelets   Q3. H. Trauma/Non accidental injury**

Q4. **G. Toxin related endothelial injury, thrombus formation, increased platelet consumption**

Q5. **D. IgA immune complex deposition in small vessels   Q6. E. Inherited bleeding tendency**

Bruising occurs most commonly following trauma. It is more severe or occurs spontaneously if there is impaired coagulation. Effective coagulation requires the presence of normal platelets and clotting factors. The pattern of bruising, duration of the history and presence of associated features may suggest the underlying cause. Our first case describes a classic episode of purpura secondary to bacterial septicaemia. Infection leads to disseminated intravascular coagulation (DIC). In DIC there is over-activation of the pathways leading to blood clotting which is generally secondary to tissue factor. This is usually expressed on subendothelium but is exposed after vessel trauma or can be induced on endothelium and mononuclear cells secondary to inflammatory mediators such as cytokines (tumour necrosis factor) or endotoxin (sepsis) (1).

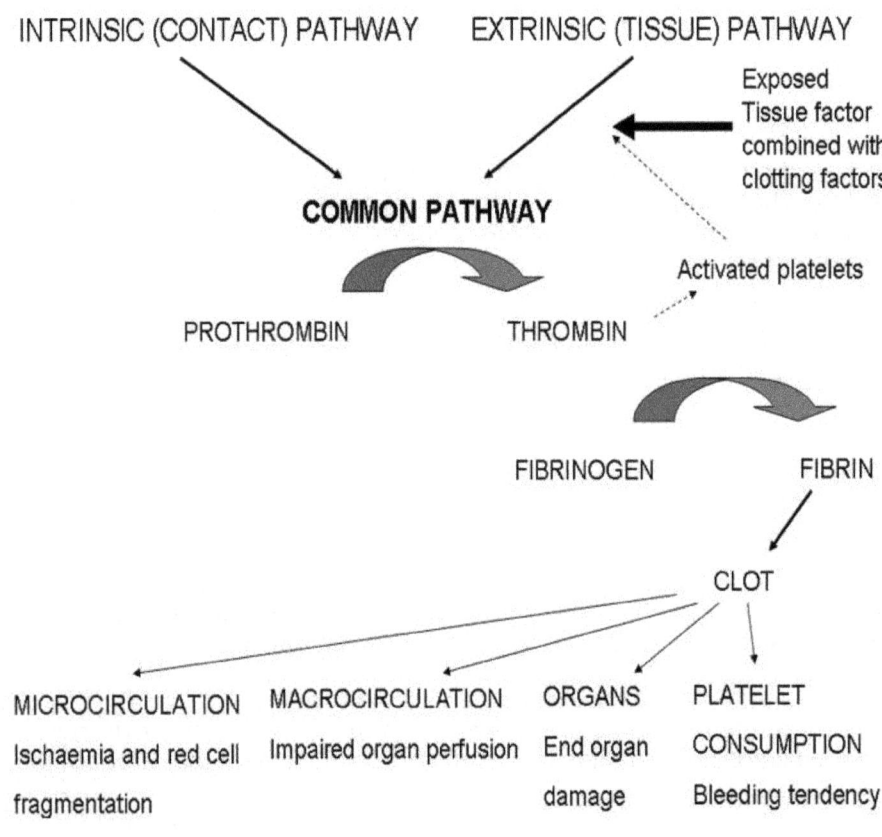

Legend: Extrinsic pathway stimulation leads to the conversion of prothrombin to thrombin. The formation of small clots leads to the consumption of clotting factors and consumption of platelets. At the same time excess circulating thrombin assists in the conversion of plasminogen to plasmin resulting in fibrinolysis. The breakdown of clots produces fibrin degradation products which have anticoagulant properties. Plasmin activates the complement and kinin systems leading to hypotension, and increased vascular permeability (1,2).

Our second case describes classic immune thrombocytopenic purpura (ITP). ITP results from IgA antiplatelet antibodies; the antibody: platelet complex is destroyed in the spleen leading to thrombocytopenia. Megakaryocyte production may also be impaired (3). It is usually a benign self limiting condition. It typically follows a viral upper respiratory tract infection in the spring or winter. A bone marrow biopsy is necessary if there are atypical features (abnormal exam, blood film abnormality). Most cases resolve spontaneously within a few weeks. Steroids suppress antibody formation and IV immunoglobulin blocks the FC receptor in the spleen reducing the rate of platelet clearance (4). Platelet transfusions are only used for acute massive haemorrhage as the platelets are destroyed by circulating antibodies. Whilst lamotrogine causes skin rashes it is valproate that often causes thrombocytopenia.

Q3. Once children become independently mobile, they are more likely to be found to have accidental bruises. However, the bruising tends to be found in certain locations. The commonest sites for accidental bruising are the knees/shins and over bony prominences. In young children, accidental bruising to the head tends to be found in a T-shape across the forehead, nose, upper lip, chin and to the back of the head (5). The presence of petechiae in association with bruising is a strong predictor of an abusive injury. The cheek and periorbital areas are uncommon sites for accidental bruises. Non accidental injury in children should always be considered. Factors which allow a judgement to be made about whether a bruise is inflicted include the plausibity of any history, medical reasons for bruising (including family history of bleeding tendencies), whether the examination findings are consistent and the overall picture (background concerns, other signs of abuse, child's demeanour).

There is no scientific evidence to support the ageing of bruising. Different people will describe the same bruise differently in terms of colour and the same individual may even describe it differently between examining the child and then reviewing the photographs. When a child presents with unexplained bruising evidence of coagulopathy should be sought. Tests should include a full blood count, clotting (APTT, PT, TT, fibrinogen), and a blood film. These tests will not exclude a platelet function problem.

The fourth case history describes haemolytic uraemic syndrome (HUS). It is characterised by microangiopathic anaemia, thrombocytopenia and renal failure. The cause is not known but HUS is associated with bacterial or viral infection of the GI tract or respiratory system. This results in endothelial injury to the microvasculature causing activation of prostaglandins and the coagulation pathway leading to the development of microthrombi. Red cells are damaged as they pass through the damaged vessels resulting in microangiopathic anaemia. Thrombocytopenia results from adhesion to the damaged vasculature, incorporation into the microthrombi, or platelet damage. There are 2 main types of HUS. The epidemic form which usually follows a gastroenteritis, typically involving bloody diarrhoea in a young child. Following this, the child will become pale and lethargic and develop dark urine and oliguria. The common causative organisms are the verotoxin-secreting form of E. Coli (E. coli 0157), Salmonella, Shigella, Campylobacter and S pneumoniae. It is commoner in the summer. The second rarer type is more sporadic and tends to be seen in older children and adults. This is less commonly associated with preceding GI infection, has a more insidious renal impairment but with more severe renal damage.

The fifth case describes Henoch Schonlein vasculitis which is an IgA-mediated small vessel vasculitis. No one is certain of the exact aetiology for HSP but IgA is deposited in the affected tissue causing an inflammatory reaction and tissue damage. The areas that are affected include skin (rash), joints (arthritis), gut (abdominal pain, intussusception) and kidneys (proteinuria, haematuria, nephritic and nephritic syndrome). The condition is commoner in males and tends to peak in winter. It may be preceded by a viral or streptococcal illness. Clinically, it often starts with an urticarial rash which progresses to a palpable purpuric rash; the rash is usually (but not exclusively) seen on the extensor surfaces of the lower limbs and buttocks. There may be associated swelling of the dorsum of the hands and feet. Renal problems, if they occur, usually manifest within the first month. Patients should be followed up for blood pressure measurements and urinalysis.

The sixth history suggests a bleeding tendency which runs through the family. Haemophilia is more likely to present with haemarthroses and deep tissue bleeding whereas von Willebrand disease (vWD) is more likely to present with easy bruising, prolonged bleeding and epistaxis. vWD is an autosomal disorder, usually inherited in a dominant manner; The abnormality is found on chromosome 12. It is characterised by a deficiency, dysfunction or absence of von Willebrand factor (vWF). vWF is necessary for the adherence of platelets to damaged endothelium; in addition, it is a carrier protein for Factor VIII protecting it from being degraded (1). Therefore depending on the deficiency of vWF (which is variable), Factor VIII may also be reduced. The bleeding time will be prolonged due to the inability of platelets to adhere to the endothelium and the APTT may be prolonged if the factor VIII level is reduced sufficiently. PT is normal. On further testing, reduction in vWF will be reduced and the riscocetin test will show a reduction in platelet aggregation relative to the

Syllabus Mapping

Haematology and oncology

- be able to interpret commonly reported clotting studies
- understand the pathophysiology of disorders of haematopoiesis, coagulation and malignancy

References

1. Chapter 11 - Disorders of coagulation; Lanzkowsky P. Manual of pediatric hematology and oncology. Elsevier 2005.

2. Morley SL. Management of acquired coagulopathy in acute paediatrics. *Arch Dis Child (E&P)* 2011; **96(2)**:49-60.

3. Scott JP, Chapter 14 - Haematology; Behrman RE, Kliegman RM. Nelson Essentials of Pediatrics. 4th ed. Philadelphia, Elsevier Saunders; 2002.

4. Gibson BES, Chapter 19 - Haematology and Oncology; Beattie J, Carachi R. Practical paediatric problems. Hodder Arnold, 2005.

5. Maguire S. Which Injuries may indicate child abuse? *Arch Dis Child* (E&P) 2010; **95(6)**:170-77.

Chapter 28: A child with anaphylaxis
Dr Sally Edwards

A 9 year old boy with no previous history of allergic reactions presents to the children's emergency department with stridor, wheeze and tachycardia. He had eaten a manufactured chocolate and nut cookie approximately 45 minutes prior to the onset of symptoms. This was the first known exposure to nuts of any kind. On arrival of the paramedics he was noted to have stridor, wheeze and tachycardia and was given intramuscular adrenaline at the scene. On arrival 12 minutes later he has inspiratory stridor, oxygen saturations of 96% (in 15L/minute of oxygen given by a mask with a reservoir bag), expiratory wheeze, a heart rate 169/minute and a blood pressure of 108/62 mmHg, there is no facial swelling nor urticaria.

Q1. Which chemical mediator is likely to be responsible for the signs and symptoms?

A.   Histamine
B.   Interleukin 4
C.   Interleukin 13
D.   Platelet activating factor
E.   Tryptase

Q2. What is the treatment you should give next?

A.   Intramuscular adrenaline
B.   Intravenous chlorphenamine
C.   Intravenous hydrocortisone
D.   Nebulised salbutamol
E.   Oral ranitidine

Answers and Rationale

Q1.   A. Histamine

Q2.   A. Intramuscular adrenaline

Anaphylaxis is a "serious life-threatening generalised or systemic hypersensitivity reaction" and a "serious allergic reaction that is rapid in onset and might cause death". Anaphylaxis is diagnosed based on clinical criteria and when any one of the following occurs on exposure to an allergen within minutes to hours:

1.   **Involvement of skin or mucosal tissue AND respiratory difficulty OR low blood pressure**

2.   **Two or more of the following**

a.   Involvement of skin or mucosa
b.   Respiratory difficulties
c.   Hypotension
d.   Gastrointestinal symptoms

3.   **Low blood pressure after exposure to a known allergen**

The World Allergy Organisation (WAO) categorises anaphylaxis as immunological i.e. IgE mediated reactions and non immunological (no immunoglobulin involvement). In allergic disease an allergen interacts with an allergen-specific IgE which is bound to the Fc epsilon RI receptor found on mast cells and/or basophils.

In atopic individuals B cells differentiate into IgE producing cells via the activity of T helper 2 cells in response to allergen exposure. This process occurs predominantly in the peripheral lymphoid tissues. In humans cytokines interleukin 4 (IL-4), interleukin 13 (IL-13) and their receptors are also contributory to IgE responses. Whilst these cytokines are important in the initial generation of antibody and can influence the degree of inflammatory cell responses they are not important mediators during an acute episode.

Surface bound IgE on mast cells and basophils interact when in close proximity to the specific allergen. Cross-linking across two or more receptors on the cell surface occurs due to either multiple identical sites for antibody binding in the allergen (multivalent) or multiple different epitopes (univalent) leading to aggregation and initiation of intracellular signalling. When this signalling is sufficiently strong the mast cells (or basophils) activate causing degranulation and mediator release. The important immediate mediators include histamine, tryptase and TNF. This then stimulates a further cascade of cytokine and mediator release and enzyme production.

These mediators either act directly on tissues or recruit and activate additional inflammatory cells particularly eosinophils.   A 'chain-reaction' of allergic inflammation is then propagated as a result of the recruited cells releasing more mediators.

The correct answer to question 1 is histamine, as histamine alone is sufficient to produce most of the symptoms of anaphylaxis. It works through the activation of both H1 and H2 receptors. H1 alone causes tachycardia, pruritis, rhinorrhoea and bronchospasm. H1 and H2 receptor activation jointly contributes to flushing, hypotension and headache. Histamine also causes coronary artery vasoconstriction increased vascular permeability.

Tryptase although abundant and relatively specific for mast cells appears to be predominantly released in response to inoculation anaphylaxis (insect stings/intravenous contrast). In our case the allergen was a food substance and tryptase only rises slightly with this and is therefore unlikely to be useful in diagnosing anaphylaxis. Nonetheless, the recent NICE guidelines remind us to take blood to check serum tryptase in all cases of suspected anaphylaxis. Beta-tryptase is the mature form of tryptase which is enzymatically active and released upon degranaulation in the secretory granules found in mast cells. It is able to activate complement, coagulation and kallikrein-kinin systems when present which contribute to hypotension, angioedema and clotting disturbances.

The role of platelet activating factor (PAF) and the enzyme which activate it have not been well defined in human anaphylaxis

With question 2, IM adrenaline is the correct answer. Adrenaline is the key medication in anaphylaxis and should be administered as soon as anaphylaxis event is suspected; a dose can be repeated after ten minutes if there are ongoing signs, as in our case. It has effects on the α, $\beta1$ and $\beta2$ receptors. Activation of the α adrenergic receptors reverses peripheral vasodilation and reduces oedema; this in turn prevents and relieves upper airway obstruction. $\beta1$ receptor activation increases the force and rate of cardiac contractions. Histamine and leukotriene release is suppressed and bronchial airways dilated through the action of $\beta2$ receptor activation.

Glucocorticoids are also useful in the management of anaphylaxis however due to the duration to the onset of action (several hours) it is unlikely to make a difference to the current episode of any scenario, although it is hoped it reduces the risk of biphasic reactions. They work by switching off transcription of activated genes that encode pro-inflammatory proteins. The Cochrane Library is unable to support or refute the advice to use them due to lack of sufficient evidence. They do potentially relieve protracted or biphasic reactions.

Antihistamines (predominantly H1 antagonists) are commonly used and are known to reduce itching, flushing, urticaria and nasal and eye symptoms. They are not believed to have an effect on airway oedema or spasm, hypotension or shock and therefore although can be considered are not going to terminate anaphylaxis in this scenario. The Cochrane Library again published a review that does not support their use in an emergency situation. The role (if any) of H2 antagonists like ranitidine in acute allergic reactions is unknown but these are sometimes useful in management of chronic spontaneous urticaria.

$\beta2$ adrenergic agonists e.g. salbutamol are sometimes given for wheezing and shortness of breath.

Although they help with lower respiratory tract symptoms they have minimal α1 adrenergic agonist vasoconstrictor effects and do not prevent or relieve laryngeal oedema, upper airway obstruction, hypotension nor shock making this answer also less correct.

Syllabus Mapping

Infection, Immunity and Allergy

• understand the scientific basis of atopy and anaphylaxis and the rationale for treatments

Pharmacology, Poisoning and Accidents

• understand the mode of action, physiological and metabolic mechanisms of therapeutic agents including intravenous fluids

References

1. Kemp, Simons, Feldweg Pathophysiology of Anaphylaxis. Uptodate Oct 2012.

2. Roger, Johnson, Stokes, Peebles. Anaphylactic Shock: Pathophysiology, Recognition and Treatment. *Semin Resp Crit Care Med* 2004;**25**:695-703.

3. Simons, et al. World Allergy Organization Guidelines for the Assessment and Management of Anaphylaxis. *Curr Opin Allergy Clin Immunol* 2012;**12**:389-99.

4. Stokes, Casale, Bochner and Feldweg. The relationship between IgE and allergic disease. *Uptodate* Oct 2012.

5. Sampson et al. Second Symposium on the definition and management of anaphylaxis: summary report – second national institute of allergy and infectious disease/food allergy and anaphylaxis network symposium. *Annals of Emerg Med* 2006;**47**:373-379.

6. NICE Anaphylaxis: assessment to confirm episode and decision to refer after emergency treatment for a suspected anaphylactic episode. NICE Clinical Guideline 134 Dec 2011.

7. Dunbar. Anaphylaxis. Postgraduate course in Paediatric Respiratory Medicine: Practical Paediatric Allergy Manual. June 2010.

Chapter 29: Varicella Zoster exposure in the newborn child Dr Benita Morrisey, Dr Arvind Shah

A community midwife calls you about a 2 day old baby girl. Her mother has just developed a rash that she suspects is chicken pox, and cannot remember whether she has had chicken pox before. She grew up in Kenya, and her own mother died a few years ago.

This is mother's first baby. She was born at 38 weeks gestation by spontaneous vaginal delivery weighing 3.65 Kg. The baby is breast-feeding well and is clinically well with no signs of chickenpox. The midwife is asking if she needs to take any action.

Q1. Which investigation result most suggests that Mother has not previously had chicken pox infection (is non-immune)?

A.   Negative maternal IgE result for Varicella Zoster virus
B.   Negative maternal IgG result for Herpes Simplex virus
C.   Negative maternal IgG result for Varicella Zoster virus
D.   Negative maternal IgM result for Varicella Zoster virus
E.   Negative PCR (polymerase chain reaction) result for Varicella zoster virus

Q2. What is the incubation period for chicken pox infection?

A.   One to three days
B.   Three to five days
C.   Five to twelve days
D.   Ten to twenty one days
E.   Fifteen to forty days

Answers and Rationale

Q1.   C. Negative maternal IgG result for Varicella Zoster virus

Q2.   D. Ten to twenty one days

Managing neonates and children with Varicella Zoster exposure or infection is a common scenario encountered in clinical practice. Varicella zoster virus is a DNA virus that causes two distinct patterns of infection. Primary varicella infection causes the diffuse vesicular rash of chicken pox. Reactivation of latent varicella zoster infection results in a more localized skin infection, herpes zoster or shingles.

Chicken pox is one of the commonest infections worldwide, and by the age of 5 around 75% of children in the UK will have had chicken pox infection. In most immunocompetent children it is a mild and self-limiting illness; however in young infants, adults and immunocompromised children it can have a much more severe course. Complications can occur however even in previously healthy children with significant morbidity and mortality.

Varicella zoster virus is a neurotropic herpes virus, similar to herpes simplex virus. It is transmitted in oropharyngeal secretions and the fluid of skin lesions either by airborne spread or direct contact. The incubation period of an infection is the time between exposure to a pathogenic organism and when symptoms and signs occur. Varicella Zoster has an incubation period of between 10-21 days, but the illness usually develops 14-16 days after exposure. During the early part of the incubation period the virus replicates in local lymphoid tissue and during a brief phase of subclinical viraemia spreads to the reticuloendothelial tissue. During a second viraemic phase, that usually lasts between 3 and 7 days, widespread cutaneous lesions occur.

Varicella zoster virus is also transmitted back to the mucosa of the upper respiratory tract and oropharynx in the late incubation period, permitting spread to susceptible contacts 1-2 days before the appearance of the rash. In immunocompetent children host immune responses limit viral replication; however in the immunocompromised child continued viral replication may lead to disseminated infection with resultant complications in the lungs, liver, brain and other organs.

Subclinical varicella infection is rare – almost all susceptible exposed contacts will go onto develop the infection. There may be prodromal symptoms of fever and malaise 24-48 hours before the rash occurs. Fever and other systemic symptoms usually resolve within 2-4 days after the onset of the rash. Varicella lesions first appear on the scalp, face or trunk; first as pruritic erythematous papules which then evolve to form clear fluid-filled vesicles. Whilst the initial lesions are crusting, new crops form on the trunk and then the extremities.

Congenital Varicella Infection

In-utero transmission of varicella can occur but is rare. Most adult women have already had chicken pox as children and are therefore immune. Congenital varicella syndrome occurs in approximately 0.4% of infants born to women who have had varicella in the 1st trimester, and around 2% of infants born to women who have had varicella between 13-20 weeks gestation. Congenital varicella syndrome is characterized by skin-scarring (in a zoster like distribution) limb hypoplasia, neurological (microcephaly, seizures and developmental delay) eye (microopthalmia, chorioretinitis, cataracts) renal (hydroureter, hydronephrosis) and autonomic nervous system abnormalities (neurogenic bladder, swallowing difficulties).

Immunoglobulins and testing for Varicella Zoster Immunity

Antibodies (immunoglobulins) are a key component of the body's specific immune system. B-lymphocytes recognize antigens (substances that induce an immune response,) and undergo antigen-mediated somatic hypermutation to become antibody-secreting plasma cells or memory cells. There are five different types or classes of immunoglobulins, and these vary in their size and biological properties, role and functional locations (Table 29.1).

Table 29.1: Summary of the properties and function of the major classes of immunoglobulin

Class	Size (kDa) (Structure)	Crosses Placenta	Normal levels mg/ml (adult)	Function
IgG	150 (Monomeric)	Yes	13	Main immunoglobulin of acquired immunity.
IgM	950 (Monomeric, Pentameric)	No	1.5	First antibody produced in response to antigen exposure, present in human serum.
IgA	160 (Monomeric, Dimeric)	No	4.5	Responsible for mucosal immunity - found in respiratory, gastro-intestinal and genito-urinary tract mucosa. Present in saliva, tears and milk.
IgD	175 (Monomeric)	No	0.03	Membrane immunoglobulin, which has role in signaling activation of B cells.
IgE	190 (Monomeric)	No	0.0001	Involved in allergic and parasitic processes. Its interaction with mast cells and basophils causes histamine release.

Immunoglobulin G (IgG) is the only antibody, which is effectively transported across the placenta, with concentrations in a full-term infant comparable to or higher than those in the mother. Much of this active transport of IgG occurs in the third trimester, so premature babies will have a much lower concentration of IgG than babies born at term. Neonates rely on maternal IgG for their first six months of life, to protect against infections, although levels start to fall rapidly after birth. Children do not attain adult levels of IgG until 7-12 years.

Other classes of antibodies are not transported across the placenta although the fetus can produce IgM and small amounts of IgA in response to intrauterine infection. Antibody tests for infection can test for both IgM and IgG antibodies to a pathogen. The IgM antibody response to an infection usually occurs earlier in the illness, and generally peaks at around 7-10 days after infection, and disappears within a few weeks. The IgG antibody response peaks at 4-6 weeks and usually persists for life. The presence of IgG antibody to a pathogen can indicate a recent seroconversion or past exposure to the pathogen. With an infection such as chickenpox, if a woman has a positive IgG antibody response to varicella zoster virus, this indicates both previous infection with and immunity to the virus.

Varicella Infection in Neonates

Mortality is particularly high in neonates born to susceptible mothers who contracted varicella around the time of birth as they do not have protective IgG antibodies against varicella zoster virus. Infants whose mothers develop varicella zoster infection in the period from 5 days prior to the delivery to 2 days after are at particularly high risk. The infant acquires the infection transplacentally as a result of maternal viraemia, which may occur up to 48 hours prior to onset of maternal rash. If a mother develops chicken pox within this high-risk period, give prophylactic zoster immunoglobulin to the newborn. If the neonate does develop chicken pox this should also be treated with intravenous aciclovir.

Syllabus Mapping

Infection, immunity and allergy
- understand host defence mechanisms and their pattern of development
- know the mechanisms of maternal to fetal transmission of infection
- know the epidemiology, pathology and natural history of common infections of childhood

Neonatology
- understand the embryology of the human fetus from conception to birth and how errors in this process can lead to diseases or congenital anomalies
- know and understand the common acquired and congenital infections in the newborn period

References

1. Chapter 34: Varicella Infection. The Green Book. Department of Health Publication. https://www.wp.dh.gov.uk/immunisation/files/2012/07/Green-Book-Chapter-34-v2_0.pdf

2. Cameron JC, Allan G, Johnston F et al. Severe complications of chickenpox in hospitalized children in the UK and Ireland. *Arch Dis Child* 2007;**92**:1062-1066.

3. Buckley RH, Chapter 117 – T Lymphocytes, B Lymphocytes and Natural Killer Cells. In; Kliegman RM, Stanton BMD, Geme J et al. Nelson Textbook of Pediatrics. 19th ed. Philadelphia, Elsevier Saunders; 2011.

4. LaRussa PS, Marin M. Chapter 245 – Varicella Zoster Virus Infections. In; Kliegman RM, Stanton BMD, Geme J et al. Nelson Textbook of Pediatrics. 19th ed. Philadelphia, Elsevier Saunders; 2011.

Suggested additional reading/resources

The Health Protection Agency offers extremely helpful advice about the duration which a child should be excluded from school/nursery following exposure to common infections including chickenpox. They suggest that children are infectious for 5 days from the onset of the rash. A single page pdf document can be accessed at the following weblink:
http://www.hpa.org.uk/webc/HPAwebFile/HPAweb_C/1194947358374

Chapter 30: Two children with rickets
Dr Nicholas Ware

Case 1

A 3 year old girl presents to the emergency department with a short history of abdominal pain and muscle weakness. On examination she is small (<2nd centile for weight and height) with frontal bossing and bowing of the legs. You suspect she may have rickets secondary to vitamin D deficiency.

Q1.   Are the following statements about vitamin D deficiency TRUE (T) or FALSE (F)?

A.   25-hydroxylation of vitamin D occurs in the liver
B.   Abdominal pain is a common presenting symptom in children
C.   Breast milk contains more vitamin D than formula milk
D.   Calcidiol is the biologically active form of vitamin D
E.   In teenagers typically less than 10% of vitamin D comes from dietary sources

As part of her initial investigations a blood gas is done which reveals she is hypocalcaemic.

Q2.   Are the following statements about hypocalcaemia TRUE (T) or FALSE (F)?

A.   Acute reduction in blood pH causes an increase in ionised calcium
B.   Cardiac arrhythmias occur typically due to QT prolongation
C.   It typically results in reduced or absent tendon reflexes
D.   It results in petechiae
E.   Laryngospasm is a recognised complication

Case 2

A 5 year old boy is referred to you from a local GP with symptoms and signs of rickets. Despite regular vitamin D supplementation he has increasing genu varum, delayed dentition and short stature. Blood tests reveal a normal calcium, low phosphate, raised alkaline phosphatase (ALP), raised parathyroid hormone (PTH) and normal vitamin D level. You suspect hypophosphataemic rickets.

Q3.   Are the following statements about hypophosphataemic rickets TRUE (T) or FALSE (F)?

A.   Approximately 25% of inherited hypophosphataemia is X-linked
B.   It is associated with glycosuria
C.   Nephrocalcinosis occurs in almost half of treated cases
D.   PTH and ALP are usually raised in all forms of rickets and are unhelpful in distinguishing between underlying causes
E.   Treatment with phosphate supplements often causes diarrhoea

Answers and Rationale

Q1.	A. False	B. True	C. False	D. False	E. True
Q2.	A. False	B. True	C. False	D. True	E. True
Q3.	A. False	B. True	C. True	D. True	E. True

Rickets occurs due to impaired mineralisation at the epiphyseal growth plate of bones and subsequent poor growth and deformity. It occurs when there is a deficiency in either calcium or phosphate, the key minerals that make up bone. The term rickets specifically applies to children where bone growth has been affected. Mineralisation defects in adults are termed osteomalacia.

Rickets presents with differing age dependent bone deformity patterns and signs. In the first year of life these include craniotabes (softening of the skull), widened sutures, frontal bossing, epiphyseal swelling (especially in the wrists), rachitic rosary (bulging costochondral joints) and a Harrison's sulcus. Older children present with genu varum or valgum, abnormal dentition, proximal myopathy and bone pain. The typical x-ray findings are of cupped and widened epiphyses, metaphysical osteopenia and Looser's zones (areas of weakness).

If vitamin D deficiency is severe enough to cause hypocalcaemia then symptoms can include paraesthesia, tetany, laryngospasm and seizures. Calcium is required for platelet function therefore hypocalcaemia can also present with easy bruising or petechiae. On examination tendon reflexes are often brisk. ECG changes include QT prolongation which may result in cardiac arrhythmia. In this situation or where seizures occur, the only effective treatment is calcium replacement, usually using intravenous preparations such as calcium gluconate.

The causes of rickets can be broadly classified as vitamin D deficiency, nutritional calcium deficiency, and renal phosphate wasting. Nutritional calcium deficiency is common in many parts of the world where calcium rich food sources are scarce (such as dairy products and green leafy vegetables). However in the UK vitamin D deficiency is more common, particularly amongst children with Asian and African backgrounds.

Vitamin D deficiency can present with the symptoms of rickets although often presents earlier with more generalised signs. The two commonest presentations in older children are abdominal pain and muscle weakness, usually with a background of growth failure. Other common symptoms include irritability, impaired concentration and hypotonia. Both nutritional calcium deficiency and vitamin D deficiency can occur as a result of gastrointestinal malabsorption and it is important to exclude this in any child presenting with any of the above signs.

It is important to understand how the metabolism of vitamin D affects bone metabolism and turnover (1-3). Overall 90% of vitamin D is synthesised in the skin by ultraviolet (UV) light. A healthy light-skinned adult will produce between 10 000 and 20 000 IU of vitamin D3 following full body exposure for 10 to 15 minutes to UV-B light in the summer months. A dark-skinned adult requires 5-10-fold this duration to synthesise a similar amount.

Whilst less than 10% typically comes from dietary sources in most of the world, UV-B levels are low in winter months in regions distant from the equator (including the UK). In these regions then dietary sources are more important. Very few foods contain much vitamin D (fatty fish livers being the exception). Breast milk is not a particularly good source of vitamin D whereas most formula milks are fortified with it and hence contain much higher concentrations. Due to the prevalence of vitamin D deficiency amongst the adult population maternal deficiency is also a significant problem with many babies being born with deficiency. The current NICE guidelines suggest that all pregnant mothers take vitamin D supplements during pregnancy (4). Healthy breastfed babies born to women who have followed this recommendation should receive vitamin D supplementation from six months of age. However if a mother is known to be vitamin D deficient or where there is uncertainty vitamin D supplements for mother and baby should be started soon after birth.

The first stage in the synthesis of vitamin D is the conversion of cholesterol to cholecalciferol by exposure to the UV rays in sunlight. Lack of sunlight is the commonest cause of vitamin D deficiency in older children (1). Cholecalciferol is then hydroxylated in the liver by the enzyme 25-alpha hydroxylase into 25-hydroxyvitamin D (calcidiol). 25-hydroxyvitamin D is then further hydroxylated in the kidney by 1-alpha hydroxylase into 1,25-dihydroxyvitamin D (calcitriol), the active form of vitamin D. Active vitamin D has a number of key roles in the metabolism of bone mineralisation. Through various receptor binding sites (including the vitamin D receptor), it promotes calcium absorption in the small intestine, promotes bone resorption via osteoclast regulation, and allows the parathyroid gland to regulate calcium and phosphate homeostasis via PTH production.

In all children presenting with rickets or signs of vitamin D deficiency it is important to measure their calcium and phosphate levels. PTH and ALP levels will be elevated in all forms of rickets reflecting the body's attempt to normalise levels through mobilisation of calcium and phosphate in bone. PTH and ALP are therefore not useful to determine the underlying cause of rickets, but are helpful markers of treatment efficacy. Vitamin D deficient children should be treated with vitamin D supplements and levels should be rechecked to ensure an effective response. Where the underlying cause is not clear both 25-hydroxyvitamin D and 1,25-dihydroxyvitamin D levels can be measured and help to isolate underlying pathology. Normal serum vitamin D levels point towards either vitamin D dependent rickets or hypophosphataemic rickets.

There are two different types of vitamin D dependent rickets, both of which are hereditary. Type 1 is due to mutations in 25-hydroxyvitamin D-1-alpha hydroxylase genes and can usually be adequately treated with 1-alpha calcidol or calcitriol. Type 2 consists of a range of vitamin D receptor defects and is characterised by early onset of severe rickets often associated with alopecia. There is currently no satisfactory treatment for type 2 although very large doses of vitamin D analogues and calcium supplements are necessary but with mixed results.

Hypophosphataemic rickets includes a number of underlying conditions including renal Fanconi syndrome (which also results in glycosuria) and oncogenic excess FGF23 production, however the commonest is X-linked dominant hypophosphataemic rickets (accounting for 80% of all inherited hypophosphataemia). This is an X-linked dominant form of vitamin D resistant rickets where vitamin D supplementation is relatively ineffective. It is a rare condition caused by a mutation in the PHEX gene sequence and treatment involves giving 1-alphacalcidol alongside phosphate supplements. To avoid large swings in serum phosphate levels supplements should be given throughout the day. In large quantities all phosphate supplements cause diarrhoea. Almost 50% of these patients develop nephrocalcinosis (5).

Syllabus Mapping

Metabolic medicine

- understand the pathophysiology of metabolic disorders e.g. electrolyte and acid base disturbance, hyperammonaemia, hypoglycaemia
- know the genetic and environmental factors in the aetiology of metabolic disorders
- know the clinical and biochemical features of electrolyte and acid base disturbances and metabolic diseases
- know the causes and investigation of metabolic bone disease
- understand the principles of dietary, vitamin and pharmacological treatment of metabolic diseases

Nutrition

- know the constituents of a healthy diet at all ages including the breast and formula feeding in infancy
- know the constitution of infant feeds commonly used in health and disease
- know the principles and methods of dietary supplementation e.g. vitamins, minerals

References

1. Wagner CL, Greer FR. Prevention of vitamin D deficiency in infants, children and adolescents. Pediatrics 2008;**122**:1142.

2. Davies J et al. Preventable but no strategy: vitamin D deficiency in the UK. *Archives of Disease in Childhood* 2011;**96(7)**:614-5.

3. Holick M. Vitamin D deficiency. *New England Journal of Medicine* 2007;**357**:266-81.

4. National Institute for Health and Clinical Excellence. (2008) *Public health guidance PH11*. Maternal and child nutrition.

5. Rees L et al. (2012). *Paediatric Nephrology*. Oxford University Press.

Chapter 31: The child with elevated ammonia
Dr Jonathan Grimbley, Dr Mark Anderson

This is a list of potential diagnoses:

A.   Glutaric aciduria type 1
B.   Maple syrup urine disease
C.   N-acetyl glutamate synthetase deficiency
D.   Ornithine transcarbamylase deficiency carrier
E.   Propionic acidaemia
F.   Transient hyperammonaemia of the newborn
G.   Very long-chain acyl-coenzyme A dehydrogenase deficiency
H.   Viral encephalitis
I.   Wilson's disease
J.   X-linked adrenoleucodystrophy
K.   Zellweger syndrome

Choose the most likely diagnosis for the following clinical scenarios. Select one answer only for each question. Each answer may be used more than once.

Q1.   A 2 year old girl is admitted with a history of lethargy for 48 hours. She had been vomiting intermittently for 24 hours and reluctant to eat or drink. She has previously had vomiting episodes requiring intravenous rehydration. Blood tests on admission reveal an ammonia of 330μmol/L (normal range 0-50μmol/L). Her blood gas and glucose are normal.

Q2.   A 5 day old girl is brought to the paediatric emergency department. She is unresponsive on admission. Investigations reveal a severe metabolic acidosis, a blood glucose of 1.4mmol/L and serum ammonia of 480μmol/L (normal range 0-100 μmol/L) and normal liver function tests. Urinalysis is positive for ketones (3+) only.

Q3.   A 4 day old girl is referred to the paediatric ward by her community midwife with poor feeding and drowsiness. Investigations reveal a severe metabolic acidosis, a blood glucose of 0.6mmol/L, a serum ammonia of 220μmol/L (normal range 0-100 μmol/L) and normal liver function tests. Urinalysis is negative for ketones, protein and leucocytes.

Answers and Rationale

Q1. D. Ornithine transcarbamylase deficiency carrier
Q2. E. Propionic acidaemia
Q3. G. Very long-chain acyl-coenzyme A dehydrogenase deficiency

In each case described the child has symptoms of, and is subsequently found to have, a high blood ammonia. As this presents with non-specific symptoms blood ammonia should be checked in all encephalopathic children. Many metabolic problems are unmasked when children are catabolic.

The Krebs cycle is fundamental to energy production in man. An acetyl group from acetyl-CoA is combined with oxaloacetate in the mitochondrion to produce citrate. Citrate then undergoes transformation back to oxaloacetate with production of carbon dioxide, guaniosine triphosphate (GTP) and the reduced forms of nicotinamide adenine dinucleotide (NADH) and ubiquinone (QH2). Reduced NADH and QH2 form the cellular energy source adenosine triphosphate (ATP). The Krebs cycle is usually driven by the conversion of glucose into pyruvate (glycolysis) and then acetyl-CoA. In catabolic states glucose is limited and other sources must be used to produce glucose or acetyl-CoA. Initially glycogen stores from liver and muscle are converted into glucose (glycogenolysis).

Once glycogen is exhausted, breakdown of protein or fatty acids is required. Protein metabolism generates pyruvate, nitrogen and other organic acids. Pyruvate is then used to produce acetyl-CoA or to produce glucose (gluconeogenesis). The nitrogen is converted into ammonia (NH3) and excreted from the body as urea. Ammonia is also derived from the gut, kidney, muscle, liver and brain (1). Ammonia in the brain is converted to neurotoxic glutamine. Ammonia is detoxified into urea via the urea cycle which comprises six hepatic enzymatic reactions. Inherited defects of these enzymes are known as the 'urea cycle disorders' (UCDs) (2). UCDs frequently present with early-onset hyperammonaemia. As the urea cycle is not essential in the production or maintenance of glucose levels hypoglycaemia is not a common presenting feature (3). The age at presentation will depend upon the enzyme involved and degree of residual enzyme activity. All the urea cycle disorders are autosomal recessively inherited except ornithine transcarbamylase (OTC) deficiency. This is X-linked recessive and presents early in male infants. Female OTC deficiency carriers are often asymptomatic but 15% have symptoms due to under-expression of OTC (2).

Fatty acid breakdown produces acetyl-CoA or succinyl-CoA which again can be used in the Krebs cycle to produce energy or can be used to make glucose via gluconeogenesis. Fatty acid oxidation produces ketones. Disorders of fatty acid oxidation (e.g. medium or very long-chain acyl-coenzyme A dehydrogenase deficiency) present during periods of catabolism with hypoglycaemia without ketosis or ketonuria and can cause hyperammonaemia due to generalised mitochondrial dysfunction. Other conditions may also cause elevated blood ammonia. Organic acidaemias (e.g. propionic acidaemia and methylmalonic acidaemia) can inhibit the production of N-acetylglutamate. Other causes of moderate to severe hyperammonaemia (ammonia concentration in excess of 200µmol/L) include transient hyperammonaemia of the newborn in preterm neonates (shunting of portal blood through the ductus venosus), Reyes syndrome and idiosyncratic reactions to drugs such as sodium valproate. (4). Mildly elevated ammonia concentrations (100-200µmol/L) are typically due to an acquired cause, for example due to liver failure, total parenteral nutrition (TPN) or sepsis, though can be found in mitochondrial disease and disorders of fatty acid oxidation. The most common cause in practice is artefactual due to delay in the sample reaching the laboratory.

The first scenario is suggestive of a UCD of which there are two listed; ornithine transcarbamylase deficiency and N-acetyl glutamate synthetase (NAGS) deficiency. NAGS deficiency is severe and presents in the early neonatal period. The age of this girl would suggest that she is an affected carrier of X-linked OTC deficiency; previous episodes of vomiting that have required hospital admission but have been dismissed as a viral illness are typical in children with late presenting OTC deficiency. Urinary orotic acid is elevated.

The second and third scenarios are similar except for the presence of ketonuria in the second scenario and lower blood glucose and ammonia concentrations in the third. The severe acidosis and hypoglycaemia make a UCD or transient hyperammonaemia of the newborn less likely and imply an impaired catabolic response, due to impaired protein or fatty acid metabolism. The absence of ketonuria in the third scenario suggests a defect of fatty acid oxidation such as very long-chain acyl-coenzyme A dehydrogenase deficiency. Fatty acid oxidation (and therefore ketone production) is not impaired in the organic acidaemias meaning propionic acidaemia is most likely in scenario two.

Figure 31.1 *A simplified diagram of the urea cycle*

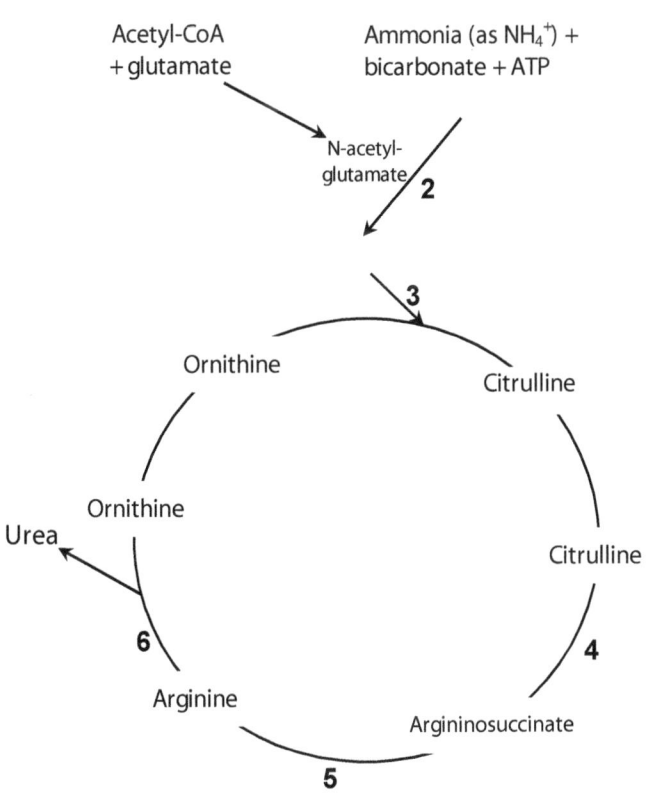

Legend: The numbers 1-6 correspond to the enzymes that catalyse the urea cycle and that may be deficient in urea cycle disorders. 1 - N-acetylglutamate synthetase; 2 - carbamylphosphate synthetase 1; 3 - ornithine transcarbamylase; 4 - argininosuccinate synthetase; 5 - argininosuccinate lyase; 6 - arginase

Syllabus Mapping

Metabolic medicine

*   understand the biochemistry of metabolism, including urea cycle, Krebs cycle
*   understand the pathophysiology of metabolic disorders, e.g. electrolyte and acid base disturbance, hyperammonaemia, hypoglycaemia
*   know the genetic and environmental factors in the aetiology of metabolic disorders
*   know the clinical and biochemical features of electrolyte and acid base disturbances and metabolic diseases

References

1. Clay AS, Hainline BE. Hyperammonaemia in the ICU. *Chest* 2007;**132**:1368-1378.

2. Walker V. Ammonia toxicity and its prevention in inherited defects of the urea cycle. *Diab Obes and Metab* 2009;**11**:823-835.

3. Haberle J, Boddaert N, Burlina A et al. Suggested guidelines for the diagnosis and management of urea cycle disorders. *Orphanet J Rare Dis* 2012;**7**:32-62.

4. Broomfield A, Grunewald S. How to use serum ammonia. *Arch Dis Child Educ Pract Ed* 2012;**97**:72-77.

Chapter 32: The boy with pointed toes
Dr Nadya James

Jacob is 22 months and his parents are worried that their son is not yet walking independently. He was born in their home country of Poland. His mother describes the delivery as 'difficult' but he was allowed home after two days of monitoring in hospital. He is generally healthy and has no developmental concerns beyond his walking. His father vaguely recalls a cousin who 'had problems' and was in a wheelchair.

In clinic Jacob crawls and pulls to stand. He will 'cruise' around furniture carefully, and with a lot of persuasion takes a couple of steps with both hands held. He has a pronounced lumbar lordosis and a waddling gait, and walks up on his tiptoes. He has good leg muscle bulk, stable hips, and equal leg length. Reflexes are reduced in the knee but not the ankle, and plantars are downgoing. There is full passive dorsiflexion at the ankles.

Q1. Which ONE of the following tests is likely to be of the most diagnostic value?

A.   Electromyography (EMG)
B.   Hip X ray
C.   MRI of the spine
D.   Muscle biopsy
E.   Serum creatine kinase

Q2. Which ONE of the following are you most likely to find on clinical examination?

A.   Decreased anal sphincter tone
B.   Decreased facial expression
C.   Macroglossia
D.   Repetitive behaviour and stereotypies
E.   Tongue fasciculation

Answers and Rationale

Q1. E. Serum creatinine kinase
Q2. C. Macroglossia

A delay in walking is a common scenario that requires a bit of diagnostic detective work to differentiate simple delay in motor skills from something more pathological. Although one of the commonest causes of late walking seen in a paediatric clinic is the benign 'familial bottom shuffler', this case suggests something more sinister is at work.

We should separate causes into neurological (upper and lower), muscular and orthopaedic. Upper motor neurone (UMN) lesions include cerebral palsy, whether hemiplegic, diplegic, quadriplegic, or dystonic/ataxic. Whilst this case history recounts a difficult birth cerebral palsy frequently occurs with no history of antenatal or perinatal problems. However, whilst clinical signs take some time to evolve clinically by 22 months we would expect him to have increased tone and reflexes in the affected limbs, and upgoing plantars. Muscle bulk may not be particularly reduced at this young age, but we would reasonably expect to find his ankles difficult to dorsiflex and for him to have a 'scissoring' gait due to stiff legs and crossed adductors. The clinical findings in Jacob do not really fit with this being an upper motor neurone problem. If it were thought UMN in origin, reasonable investigations could include an MRI scan of the brain, and also hip X-ray at around 30 months of age to check for dislocation.

Lower motor neurone (LMN) lesions can be due to trauma/anatomical disease (such as spina bifida or a spinal tumour) or due to a generalised disease (such as spinal muscular atrophy). Spina bifida has declined since the discovery of the value of periconceptual folic acid, and antenatal ultrasound has now helped to identify many cases early. A spinal lesion would produce a combination of leg weakness and low tone, reduced/absent leg reflexes, and muscle wasting. Fasciculations, which can be seen clinically or on electromyography (EMG), are a feature of LMN disease. If the spinal cord or cord roots are involved, you would look carefully for involvement of the sacral nerve roots S1 to S4, as these govern continence and sphincter control. Anal sphincter tone can be assessed by gently pulling apart the buttocks, and anal reflexes by stroking the perianal margin. The upper limbs and rest of the body would be unaffected unless the lesion was much higher, and cervical or thoracic spina bifida is usually clinically more severe than the commoner lumbar type.

Spinal muscular atrophy (SMA) is an autosomal recessive disease, and the gene codes for an important protein called SMN1, which is involved in motor neuron survival. SMA causes progressive degeneration of the alpha motor neuron from anterior horn cells in the spinal cord. Progressive LMN weakness occurs in all muscles, most notable the proximal muscles rather than the distal. If Jacob had SMA, he would have a more global weakness/hypotonia, with very reduced/absent reflexes in his extremities. We might also see tongue fasciculation. The diagnostic test for SMA would be genetic.

Returning to the questions: Toe walking would not be a recognised feature of a LMN lesion, and Jacob's good muscle bulk and normal ankle reflexes are against him having a significant LMN problem. Electromyography is thus unlikely to be of help in his diagnosis, and we would not expect to find tongue fasciculation or decreased anal sphincter tone on examination.

Muscular disorders include problems at the neuromuscular junction (myasthenia gravis) and those of the muscle fibres themselves (muscular dystrophy). Myasthenia gravis is an autoimmune disorder where antibodies are directed against acetylcholine (ACh) nicotinic postsynaptic receptors at the neuromuscular junction. This leads to a reduced number of receptors available to be activated by release of ACh from the presynaptic LMN. The classic symptoms are of fatigable weakness, with successive LMN impulses generating ever weaker muscle contractions. The presenting symptoms are commonly of eye lid weakness, decreased facial expression, bulbar symptoms (speech and swallowing problems), and of muscle weakness (proximal more than distal, upper limb more commonly that lower). Fortunately, heart and smooth muscle have different structure ACh receptors and are not affected. The typical pattern is with weakness getting worse throughout an activity, and recovering with rest. Many patients find the weakness worse if they are hot and better if they are cooled (for example having a cold shower). Physical exam may show ptosis and rapid fatigability. Tendon reflexes and plantars would be normal, and you would not expect the child to be walking on their toes as is described in the vignette. Diagnosis of myasthenia gravis can be aided by antibody testing, electromyography, or administration of the anticholinesterase edrophonium and assessing the improvement in muscle strength caused by the resultant increase in ACh at the neuromuscular junction (the tensilon test).

Duchene muscular dystrophy is one of a group of muscular dystrophies leading to progressive loss of muscle fibres. Inheritance is X-linked recessive and females are unaffected carriers. The dystrophin gene codes for a large protein that is important in sarcolemmal stability. Without this, muscle fibres are repeatedly damaged over time and eventually necrosed fibres are replaced by fat and connective tissue. As a result, a muscle can look deceptively healthy or even hypertrophied, but be very abnormal under the microscope. Clinical symptoms start with proximal muscle weakness, which can manifest with delayed walking. Children are adaptable, and may overcome a difficulty in getting from the floor to standing by holding onto furniture. The well-known version of this is the Gower sign, where a child gets from prone lying to standing through a series of manoeuvres to overcome the weak hip muscles. Other clinical findings would include the calf hypertrophy mentioned above, and a 'waddling' gait with a lumbar lordosis. The child will often walk on their toes although the ankle is flexible (tendon shortening and contractures may develop later). Interestingly, although plantars are down-going and ankle reflexes are usually present, knee reflexes may be absent. The archetypal finding is of calf hypertrophy, and it is well recognised that patients may also have macroglossia.

Looking back at Jacob, the boy in the vignette, he has findings consistent with Duchene muscular dystrophy. A useful investigation would be to measure creatinine kinase, as this is elevated due to ongoing muscle damage. A positive result could be confirmed on genetic testing.

Orthopaedic problems leading to late walking include developmental dysplasia of the hip, which may be revealed by asymmetric skin creases, apparent femoral shortening (the Galeazzi test), or limited hip abduction in flexion. Neurology and ankle exam will be normal. Although ultrasound is used to diagnose this in infants less than 4 months of age, hip X-ray is used above this age.

Syllabus Mapping

Musculoskeletal

- understand the pathophysiological changes which occur in muscle and joint disorders
- know the genetic and environmental factors in the aetiology of musculoskeletal disorders
- know the investigations used in the diagnosis of musculoskeletal disorders

Neurology and neurodisability

- know the current theories of the pathophysiology of neurodevelopmental disorders, including cerebral palsy
- understand the physiological and pathophysiological changes that occur in neurological disorders
- understand the scientific basis of normal and disordered neurodevelopment in childhood

References

1. Gupta and Appleton. Cerebral palsy: not always what it seems. *Arch Dis Child* 2001;**85**:356–360.

2. Purves D, Augustine GJ, Fitzpatrick D, et al., editors. Neuroscience. 2nd edition. Sunderland (MA): Sinauer Associates; 2001. Damage to Descending Motor Pathways: The Upper Motor Neuron Syndrome.

3. Purves D, Augustine GJ, Fitzpatrick D, et al., editors. Neuroscience. 2nd edition. Sunderland (MA): Sinauer Associates; 2001. The Lower Motor Neuron Syndrome.

4. Chaplais and McFarlane. A review of 404 'late walkers'. *Arch Dis Child* 1984;**59**:512-516.

5. Symons A, Townsend G and Hughes T. Dental characteristics of patients with Duchenne muscular dystrophy. ASDC Journal of dentistry for children.

Chapter 33: A teenager with unusual signs
Dr Richard Hastings

You see a 15 year old girl in the emergency department. They have a GP referral letter:

I would be most grateful if you could see this girl who presents with a two week history of back pain. This morning she developed weakness and numbness of her left leg. Currently she has normal bladder and bowel function but reduced power to her left leg. Knee and ankle jerk reflexes are absent. She reports reduced sensation to her left leg below the knee.

You examine the girl. She looks well and you find no abnormalities with her respiratory or cardiovascular systems. Her abdominal examination is normal. She has pain on palpation of her spine in the lower-thoracic region. Neurology is normal in her upper limbs and right leg. Her left leg shows increased tone and reduced power (3/5 or 4/5 on the MRC power scale) for hip abduction and all movements of her knee, ankle and toes. You are unable to elicit her knee and ankle deep tendon reflexes despite trying several reinforcement techniques. Plantar reflex is equivocal. She has paraesthesia to her thigh and near absent sensation to fine touch, pain and temperature below this. Proprioception to her great toe is also absent.

Q1. How would you investigate this patient?

A.   Chest X-ray
B.   CT head and spine
C.   Electromyography (EMG)
D.   MRI brain and spine
E.   No investigation

Q2. Concerning the sensory pathways which of the following statements is TRUE or FALSE?

A.   Hemisection of the spinal cord would cause contralateral loss of fine touch and proprioception
B.   Her symptoms suggest a lesion to the right side of her spinal cord
C.   The dorsal column tracts decussate in the brain stem
D.   The sensory neuronal pathways are mostly composed of two neurons
E.   The spinothalamic tract carries pain and temperature sensation

Q3. Regarding the motor neuron pathways which of the following statements is TRUE or FALSE?

A.   Areflexia is a sign of LMN lesion
B.   Hemisection of the spinal cord causes contralateral paralysis
C.   Hypertonia is a sign of an upper motor neuron (UMN) lesion
D.   Poliomyelitis affecting right-sided anterior horn cells never causes left sided weakness
E.   The cell body of the lower motor neuron (LMN) is in the medulla

Answers and Rationale

Q1: E. No investigation

Q2: A. False	**B. False**	**C. True**	**D. False**	**E. True**
Q3: A. True	**B. False**	**C. True**	**D. True**	**E. False**

No investigations are warranted since this child's signs do not fit with an organic pathology. When thinking about a potential neurological lesion you must always consider where the problem is likely to arise within the nervous system and to do this you must know the anatomy of both motor and sensory pathways. Not only will this give you clues as to the type of pathology you are seeing but it can also identify those children who have non-organic pathology. The child detailed above has incongruous signs. Firstly, she has both UMN and LMN signs and secondly, she has a pattern of sensory loss which does not fit with the anatomy of the sensory neuronal pathways. Whilst some forms of demyelination can present with a mixture of upper and lower motor neuron signs such incongruity should prompt a discussion with a neurologist before embarking upon investigation.

Sensory pathways

Sensory pathways are composed of primary, secondary and tertiary neurons (1). Primary neurons take signals from receptors (e.g. nociceptors, proprioceptors) to synapse with secondary neurons in the central nervous system. Secondary sensory neurons pass from the spinal cord or brain stem to the thalamus where they synapse with tertiary neurons. Along their path all secondary neurons decussate (cross over to the contralateral side relative to the stimulant) but the place where they decussate varies according to the type of sensory neuron (see below). Tertiary neurons conduct impulses from the thalamus to the primary somatosensory area of the cerebral cortex on the post-central gyrus.

Sensory impulses for fine touch, vibration and proprioception travel in the dorsal columns of the spinal cord. The primary neurons for these sensory modalities synapse with secondary neurons in the medulla and only then do they decussate. This means their path in the spinal cord is ipsilateral to the stimulant. In contrast, primary neurons for pain and temperature sensation enter the spinal cord and immediately synapse with secondary neurons in the dorsal horn of grey matter. These secondary neurons decussate in the spinal cord within 1-2 spinal segments then pass upwards. Therefore, unlike the sensation of fine touch, vibration and proprioception the impulses of pain and temperature sense travel up the spinal cord to the thalamus on the contralateral side to the stimulant. The result of this is that hemisection of the spinal cord can cause ipsilateral loss of fine touch and proprioception, ipsilateral paralysis and contralateral loss of pain and temperature sensation (Brown-Sequard syndrome). In the clinical case our teenager's signs are all on the left side - but it would be near impossible to have a lesion in the spinal cord which could affect the left dorsal column and the right spinothalamic tract.

Most sensory impulses for the face (touch, temperature, pain and proprioception) travel via cranial nerve V (trigeminal; a primary neuron) to synapse in the pons with secondary neurons. Secondary neurons decussate in the pons and send impulses to the thalamus in the contralateral trigeminothalamic tract.

Tertiary neurons travel from the thalamus to the primary somatosensory area of the cerebral cortex.

Motor pathways

In simple terms, pathways giving voluntary control of skeletal muscle are composed of upper and lower motor neurons. The nerves directly innervating skeletal muscle are LMNs. Most upper motor neurons pass voluntary impulses from the cerebral cortex to synapse with LMNs (either indirectly via interneurons or directly). Other pathways innervating LMNs include those from basal nuclei and the cerebellum. The majority of signals controlling the limbs and trunk are carried by UMNs in the corticospinal tracts. These pathways decussate in the medulla and synapse with LMNs in the anterior horn of the spinal cord. Therefore UMN lesions above the medulla lead to contralateral paralysis (e.g. cerebral palsy) whereas when the UMN is affected below the medulla or if the LMN is affected then an ipsilateral lesion occurs (e.g. poliomyelitis).

Cranial nerves (with motor function) are examples of lower motor neurons. From the cerebral cortex, UMNs pass down the corticobulbar tracts to synapse with the cranial nerves in motor nuclei found in the brain stem. Some of these UMNs decussate but others do not – so there is bilateral innervation of many cranial nerves. This phenomenon leads to sparing of muscles for facial expression in the upper part of the face with an UMN lesion (but not with a LMN lesion such as Bell's palsy).

Lesions affecting LMNs cause flaccid paralysis with areflexia because there is loss of all innervation to the muscle. With an UMN lesion there is loss of both voluntary and involuntary inhibitory signals from higher centres. This can lead to increased (unopposed) reflexes and hypertonia. So for example, when the bladder fills a reflex leads to contraction of the bladder wall but voluntary signals normally inhibit this contraction (until we get to a toilet). An UMN lesion will lead to loss of these inhibitory signals and the bladder will contract uncontrollably causing urinary incontinence (2). In our clinical case above our teenager has both LMN signs (arreflexia) and UMN signs (increased tone) – both of these signs are relatively easy to simulate. By understanding the anatomy of the motor and sensory tracts you can avoid further investigation of this child for a spinal cord lesion and focus on giving her any other help/support she may need.

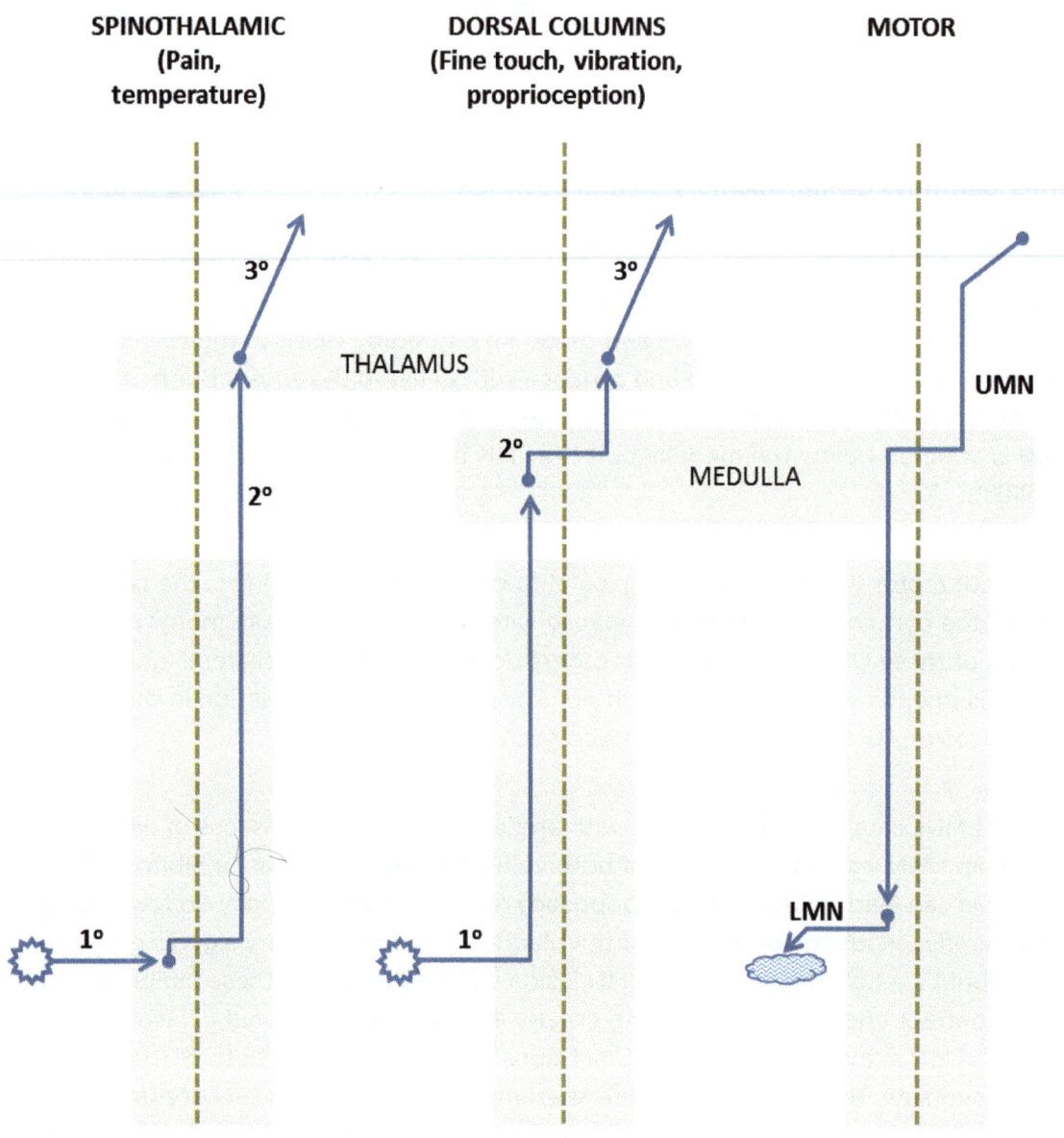

Syllabus Mapping

Neurology and neurodisability

- know the anatomy and understand the physiology of the central and peripheral nervous systems.

References

1. Monkhouse WS. Master Medicine, Clinical Anatomy. 2nd ed. Edinburgh: Churchill Livingstone; 2007.

2. Tortora GJ, Derrickson BH. Principles of Anatomy and Physiology International Student Version. 13th ed. Hoboken, N.J: John Wiley & sons; 2011.

Chapter 34: A teenager with persistent headache Dr Maria Moran, Dr Will Carroll

A 15 year old girl is referred to paediatric outpatients with a history of chronic headache over the last 6 weeks. She has been taking paracetamol and ibuprofen regularly for the headache without much relief. The headache is there most mornings when she wakes up with between a 5 and 10 severity. Any activity particularly bending over makes it worse. She has started to miss some school because of the headache. She has not noticed any visual disturbance. There is no past medical history of note.

On examination her BMI is 31. She is alert and answering questions appropriately. She is noted to have bilateral papilloedema. Neurological and systemic examinations are otherwise unremarkable. An urgent MRI head scan shows no obvious structural abnormality. She goes on to have a lumbar puncture which shows an opening pressure of 35cm H_2O (upper limit of normal 20cm H_2O) but the CSF was clear and colourless with no cells or organisms found on microscopy.

Each of the following stems may be either true or false. For the following questions which are true and which are false?

Q1.   If her symptoms continue as described above, the following treatments are likely to be effective

A.   Acetazolamide
B.   Furosemide
C.   Hypoventilation
D.   Lying flat in a quiet room
E.   Reduction in CSF volume by lumbar puncture

Q2.   When investigating new drug options for use in neurological disease, drugs that reach the brain easily from the circulation have the following molecular characteristics:

A.   Able to bind to transport receptors
B.   Highly charged
C.   Lipophilic
D.   Protein structures of similar size to plasma proteins
E.   Small non-polar

Answers and Rationale

Q1. **A. True** **B. True** **C. False** **D. False** **E. True**
Q2. **A. True** **B. False** **C. True** **D. False** **E. True**

The symptoms and signs described in the case are those of raised intracranial pressure (ICP). The body will try to keep intracranial pressure constant and as the volume of the skull is relatively fixed past infancy this pressure is determined by the volume of its contents: blood, cerebrospinal fluid (CSF), the brain itself and any pathological structure. If the volume of any of these contents increases, there is some limited ability to compensate by decreasing the volume of the others where possible. Manoeuvres such as hyperventilation rapidly but transiently reduce cerebral blood flow and therefore reduce ICP. Gravity (and therefore body position) influences a range of organ systems (1). The normal pressure in the cerebrospinal fluid (CSF) system when lying in a horizontal position varies between 6 and 20 cm CSF in a healthy adult. Variations in pressure depend on the position of the body and the pressure can be negative (lower than the atmospheric pressure) in a standing position. In patients with intracranial hypertension it is common practice to elevate the head of the bed to 30 degrees. This may restore a normal ICP when elevated via changes in several parameters including mean arterial pressure, central venous pressure and CSF displacement. A suspicion of raised ICP needs urgent evaluation, whether it is acute or chronic, because of the serious nature of conditions which cause it (see below).

Table 34.1: *Causes of raised intracranial pressure and possible treatments in children*

Pathology affecting	Example of condition	Possible treatments
Blood	Intracranial bleed (extradural) Obstructed venous drainage Blood flow ie hypertension	Surgery (if accessible) Anticoagulation (clexane) Antihypertensives
CSF	Hydrocephalus: obstructive or communicating	Surgery (shunt) Gravity
Brain	Trauma causing oedema Inflammation (encephalitis/ADEM) Encephalopathy	Mannitol Fluid restriction Steroids
Other structure	Tumour or abscess	Antibiotics Steroids Chemotherapy
None of the above	Idiopathic intracranial hypertension	Carbonic anhydrase inhibitors CSF withdrawal

Raised ICP is suggested by a combination of headache, vomiting and papilloedema although it presents may arise from the effect of pressure on the optic nerve and include visual field defects. A sixth nerve palsy may lead to diplopia. This "false-localising" sign of raised ICP occurs because the sixth nerve has the longest intracranial course of any of the cranial nerves making it particularly vulnerable to stretching and/or compression.

In our clinical case the brain appears structurally normal but CSF opening pressure is elevated. This suggests a diagnosis of idiopathic intracranial hypertension (IIH). IIH is a rare condition, more commonly seen in obese females. Case series have shown a more equal sex distribution in younger children. In recent UK studies 60% of cases were obese (2). The pathophysiology of IIH is still unclear. To understand the possible treatments used in IIH it helps to remember the physiology of CSF production and flow.

CSF is mostly produced by the choroid plexuses: these blood vessels protrude into the ventricles of the brain. The epithelial cells of the plexus have a number of ion transporters which act to provide a net movement of sodium, chloride and bicarbonate ions into the CSF, which draw water with them by osmosis (3). Most CSF production is in the lateral ventricles. From here it passes into the third ventricle and through the aqueduct of Sylvius into the fourth ventricle. It leaves the fourth ventricle to enter the cisterna magna and then flows around the brain in the subarachnoid space. This is enclosed by the arachnoid mater whose projections into the venous sinuses are called arachnoid villi which return CSF into the venous circulation. Around 500mls of CSF are produced each day in the adult, meaning the entire CSF volume will be secreted and reabsorbed between 3-4 times each day.

IIH treatment relies on reducing CSF volume, either through reducing production or improving drainage (4). Weight loss is also beneficial in overweight patients. Draining CSF at the initial lumbar puncture (or on repeat LPs) to leave a normal CSF pressure can also provide lasting relief in some patients. First line medical treatment is usually acetazolamide, a carbonic anhydrase inhibitor (5). Carbonic anhydrase inhibition with acetazolamide causes a decrease in production of CSF of up to 60%. Additional reduction of CSF production can be achieved by using furosemide. Furosemide is an inhibitor of the Na/K/2Cl carrier in the renal tubules acting as a loop diuretic. This carrier is also present in the choroid plexus epithelium, although clinically furosemide may act to reduce intracranial pressure more through its weak carbonic anhydrase inhibiting properties and its diuretic action which decrease total body extracellular water. More recently topiramate has been used, more details on the pharmacology of topiramate can be found in chapter 42. It also partially inhibits carbonic anhydrase and can cause weight loss through appetite suppression making it a potentially useful drug in IIH. Non-medical treatments (surgery including ventriculo-peritoneal shunts or transverse sinus stenting) for IIH focus on improving drainage of CSF (6).

Drugs and the blood-brain barrier: The brain is generally well protected from substances in the systemic circulation through physiological blood-brain (BBB) and blood-CSF "barriers". These barriers are formed by special tight junctions between the endothelial cells of the brain and choroid plexus capillaries which prevent easy diffusion of solutes and larger molecules between the cells. Thus to enter the brain or CSF substances must pass through rather than between cells. The cell membrane contains phospholipids so lipid-soluble (or lipophilic) molecules like ethanol, oxygen and carbon dioxide can cross this by simple diffusion. Smaller, non-polar molecules are generally more lipid soluble. However charged or polar molecules require facilitated diffusion or active transport through a protein channel. The endothelium has special transport proteins for specific nutrients needed by the brain, for example GLUT-1 for glucose and transferrin receptors for iron. Plasma proteins and large non-lipid-soluble organic molecules do not cross into the brain or CSF easily, if at all. This makes finding drug treatments to reach the CNS in adequate concentrations very difficult. It is a problem for most antibiotics, although in CNS infection such as meningitis the integrity of the BBB is affected by inflammation so drugs which normally do not cross, such as penicillin, are able to enter in sufficient concentrations. Higher doses of drugs may be needed to achieve clinically useful concentrations of drugs. This is true of acetazolamide which is usually protein-bound and used in relatively high doses to achieve effect in IIH. Sometimes direct injection of drugs into the CNS may be needed, for example, intrathecal injection of methotrexate in the treatment of leukaemia. The BBB can help a drug's mechanism of action. Mannitol is one such drug. It is a sugar alcohol which acts as an osmotic diuretic. When given intravenously it forms an osmotic gradient which draws water from the extracellular space into the circulation, and is then filtered but not reabsorbed by the kidney, causing a diuresis. It is used in the emergency treatment of acutely raised intracranial pressure because of this osmotic action, which relies on an intact BBB. Because mannitol must be given intravenously, it is reserved for emergency treatment of raised ICP usually with a deteriorating conscious level; it is not used as a regular medication for chronic symptoms so is not a very useful treatment in IIH.

Syllabus Mapping

Pharmacology, Poisoning and Accidents:

- understand the mode of action, physiological and metabolic mechanisms of therapeutic agents including intravenous fluids
- understand the planned and undesired effects of therapeutic agents

Neurology and Neurodisability

- know the anatomy and understand the physiology of the central and peripheral nervous systems
- understand the physiological and pathophysiological changes that occur in neurological disorders including raised ICP and IIH
- understand the pharmacology of agents commonly used in neurological disease including antiepileptic drugs

References

1. Martin-Du Pan, RC, Benoit R, Girardier L. The role of body position and gravity in the symptoms and treatment of various medical diseases. *Swiss Med Wkly* 2004;**134**:543–551.

2. Matthews YY, et al. UK surveillance of childhood idiopathic intracranial hypertension. *Arch Dis Child* 2012;**97**:A6.

3. Brown PD et al. Molecular mechanisms of cerebrospinal fluid production. *Neuroscience* 2004;**129**(4):957-970.

4. Biousse V, et al. Update on the pathophysiology and management of idiopathic intracranial hypertension. *J Neurol Neurosurg Psychiatry* 2012;**83**:488-494.

5. Matthews YY. Drugs used in childhood idiopathic or benign intracranial hypertension. *Arch Dis Child Educ Pract Ed* 2008;**93**:19-25.

6. Bussiere M, et al. Unilateral transverse sinus stenting of patients with idiopathic intracranial hypertension. *Am J Neuroradiol* 2010;**31**:645-50.

Chapter 35: A baby with a hole in the heart
Dr Gitika Joshi, Dr Demetris Taliotis

An 8 week old infant is noted to be tachypnoeic during routine 8 week baby check. Mum is 25 years of age and has learning difficulties. She reports that the child has a "cold" and is a bit off feeds. On examination he has a respiratory rate of 70 per minute, oxygen saturations of 95% in air, with mild subcostal recession. A loud 3/6 pansystolic murmur is heard in the left lower sternal edge which radiates to the apex. A liver edge is felt 1 cm below the costophrenic margin. An echocardiogram is performed and confirms a moderate size subaortic perimembranous ventricular septal defect (VSD).

Q1. Which ONE of the following BEST predicts the degree of Heart Failure?

A.   Degree of cyanosis
B.   Intensity of murmur
C.   Pulmonary: Aortic flow ratio (Qp:Qa)
D.   Systolic: Diastolic blood pressure ratio
E.   VSD size

Q2. On echocardiogram what changes may you expect in this child with Moderate size VSD? Mark as True (T) or False (F)

A.   Dilation (volume loading) of the left atrium
B.   Dilation (volume loading) of the left ventricle
C.   Dilation (volume loading) of the right atrium
D.   Dilation (volume loading) of the right ventricle
E.   Hypertrophy of the left ventricle
F.   Hypertrophy of the right ventricle

Q3. Which types of VSD are likely to close spontaneously? True (T) or False (F)

A.   Moderate apical VSD
B.   Moderate inlet VSD
C.   Moderate muscular VSD
D.   Moderate outlet VSD
E.   Small perimembranous VSD

Q4. What is the best indicator for early corrective surgery?

A.   Aortic valve regurgitation in a perimembranous VSD
B.   Evidence of cardiac failure
C.   Failure to thrive
D.   Left atrial enlargement
E.   Size of the VSD

Answers and Rationale

Q1. **C. Pulmonary: Aortic flow Ration (Qp:Qa)**

Q2.	A. True	B. True	C. False	D. False	E. False	F. False
Q3.	A. True	B. False	C. True	D. False	E. True	

Q4. **A. Aortic valve regurgitation in a perimembranous VSD**

Ventricular septal defects (VSD) are holes between the right and left ventricle which enable blood to escape from the left ventricle to the right creating an excessive blood flow in the pulmonary circulation. Symptoms depend on the degree of the pulmonary overcirculation. The shunt is typically left to right and the child is pink.

The magnitude of shunt depends on: 1. the size of the defect and 2. the pulmonary vascular resistance (PVR). In a small VSD, most resistance to flow occurs at the site of defect and the magnitude of the left to right shunt is small. There is gradual reduction in the PVR in newborns, from systemic levels at birth to physiological levels by 6-8 weeks. In larger defects the resistance offered by the defect is low. Here the magnitude of the shunt depends on the PVR and the symptoms start to develop as PVR falls at 6 to 8 weeks. If the defect is able to limit the transmission of pressure from the left to the right side of the heart, it is called a restrictive defect (1). The magnitude of the shunt produced by a VSD is described by the ratio of the pulmonary (Qp) to systemic (Qs) blood flow. The Qp:Qs ratio is over 1.5:1 for moderate defects and over 2:1 for large defects. Symptoms of heart failure are usually present at this level and the Qp:Qs ratio is the best predictor of failure (2).

The left to right shunt in VSDs occurs mainly in systole, when the right ventricle (RV) is contracted and the pulmonary valve is open. As a result the shunted blood goes directly into the pulmonary artery rather than remain in the RV cavity. Thus, there is no significant volume loading of the RV. The shunt through the VSD increases the pulmonary blood flow and in turn increases the pulmonary venous return to the left atrium and ventricles. Hence the chambers that dilate due to excessive left to right shunt and volume loading in a large VSD are the left atrium and left ventricle (1).

If a significant VSD is left untreated then chronic pulmonary hypertension occurs which leads to irreversible pulmonary veno-occlusive disease. This in turn leads to reversal of the shunt at ventricular level from right to left and to progressive cyanosis (Eisenmenger's Syndrome). Perhaps surprisingly, the signs of heart failure will reduce as pulmonary overcirulation reduces (3).

Embryologically, closure of the intraventricular foramen is dependent upon three factors: continued growth of connective tissue on the crest of the muscular septum; downward growth of ridges dividing the conus; and projections into the atrioventricular (AV) canal from the right-sided endocardial cushions. Since these multiple factors are involved in closure of the region encompassing the membranous septum, it is not unexpected that the most common defect occurs at this site.

There are four basic anatomic types of VSD based upon their location on the ventricular septum which can be divided into four areas:

1. Inlet muscular septal defects (8% of VSDs) : these are inferoposterior to the perimembranous defects. They are found in the area between the annulus of the tricuspid valve and the attachments of the

tricuspid valve to the RV wall.

2. Outlet or sub pulmonary muscular septal defects (5-7% of VSDs): The outlet or infundibular septum extends up to the pulmonary valve from the trabecular area.

3. Trabecular Muscular Septal Defects (5-20% of VSDs): These extend from the inlet area out to the apex and incorporate the coarse, trabeculated area of the right ventricle. Apical defects can be difficult to visualize on echocardiography due to their position and being surrounded by heavily trabeculated muscle.

4. Perimembranous Septal Defects (70-80% of VSDs): Occur at the intersection between the trabecular, inlet, and outlet areas. They are commonly partially covered by the septal leaflet of the tricuspid valve on the right site (4).

Figure 35.1. Positions of different types of VSD

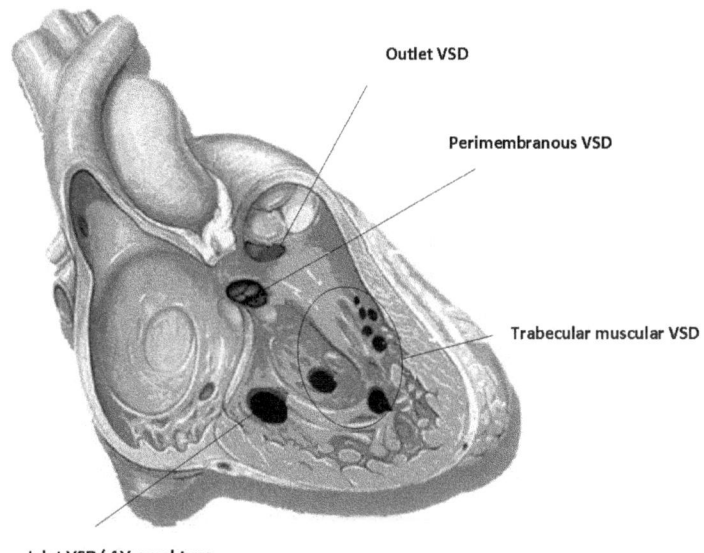

The natural history of VSDs includes spontaneous closure of the majority of small defects in the first few years of life. In general, small and moderate sized perimembranous and apical trabecular VSDs tend to close spontaneously whilst moderate inlet and outlet defects are less likely to do so. Large defects of any type are less likely to close. For those which remain patent surgical correction by 1 year of age reduces the risk of pulmonary hypertension. As a bridge to surgery children with moderate to large VSDs often have cardiac failure treated medically.

Diuretics - Furosemide and spironolactone decrease the amount of fluid in the circulation. By doing so they also reduce the volume of blood pumped across the pulmonary circulation.
ACE Inhibitors- (eg Captopril, Enalapril) act as weak diuretics as well as systemic vasodilators, reducing the systemic vascular resistance (SVR), and therefore allowing blood to be diverted from the pulmonary into the systemic circulation.
Digoxin- is a weak inotropic agent which may be indicated if diuretics and ACE inhibitors alone are not enough to control the cardiac failure.

If medical treatment is not sufficient to control the cardiac failure, and the child is unsuitable for full surgical repair (too small, or inaccessible VSD), then pulmonary artery banding can be performed. This involves placing a restrictive band around the main pulmonary artery to control the amount of blood flow to the lungs.

The size of the VSD is a poor guide to whether surgery is indicated as even large VSDs in the perimembranous septum can become restrictive or even close with time as tricuspid valve tissue grows around the defect. Whilst left atrial and ventricular volume loading is indicative of the amount of left to right shunt, and though it may indicate the need for medical treatment or pulmonary artery banding it is not an indication for early corrective surgery. Early corrective surgery is however sometimes indicated in perimembranous VSDs due to aortic valve prolapse into the VSD. This can lead to progressive aortic valve regurgitation, causing permanent damage to the aortic valve. The Bundle of His is related to the posterior inferior quadrant of a perimembranous defect and the superior anterior quadrant of inlet muscular defects hence these defects are associated with conduction abnormalities. The aortic valve cusp can herniate through infundibular and perimembranous defects leading to aortic regurgitation. Children with VSDs are at increased risk of infective endocarditis.

Syllabus Mapping

Cardiology

*   understand the pathophysiology of cardiac conditions, including cyanosis, heart failure, shock, syncope and unexpected cardiac death
*   be able to select and interpret appropriate investigations in a child with suspected cardiac pathologies

References and Further Reading

1. Myung K.Park. Paediatric Cardiology for Practitioners, 5th Ed. Mosby 2008. Pages 127-129 & 166-174.

2. Driscoll DJ. Left-To-Right Shunt Lesions. *Pediatr Clin North Am* 1999;**46**:355-368.

3. Galie N, et al. Management of pulmonary arterial hypertension associated with congenital systemic-to-pulmonary shunts and Eisenmenger's syndrome. *Drugs* 2008;**68(8)**:1049-66.

4. Van Praagh R, Geva T, Kreutzer J. Ventricular septal defects: how shall we describe, name and classify them? *J Am Coll Cardiol* 1989;**14(5)**:1298-9.

5. Litwin SB. Colour atlas of congenital heart surgery. Mosby 1996.

Chapter 36: A grunting baby
Dr Balasubramaniam

A baby is born at 29 weeks gestation by spontaneous vaginal delivery. Soon after birth the baby was noted to be grunting with subcostal and intercostal recession.

Q1.   Regarding neonatal respiratory distress which ONE of the following statements concerning grunting is most correct? It:

A.   Increases endogenous surfactant production
B.   Increases the critical closing volume
C.   Increases the functional residual capacity
D.   Is an inspiratory sound due to narrowing of the glottis
E.   Reduces the residual volume

The baby gradually deteriorates and is intubated and ventilated. Surfactant is administered through the endotracheal tube.

Q2.   Which of the following statements regarding exogenous surfactant are TRUE or FALSE in a neonate with respiratory distress syndrome? It:

A.   Improves lung compliance
B.   Improves oxygenation and ventilation
C.   Increases alveolar surface tension
D.   Maintains residual lung volume
E.   Reduces the critical closing volume

Answers and Rationale

Q1. **C. Increases the functional residual capacity**
Q2. **A. True** **B. True** **C. False** **D. True** **E. True**

Respiratory distress syndrome (RDS) occurs mostly in premature infants and its incidence is inversely proportional to gestational age and birth weight (1-3). It occurs in 60-80% of infants less than 28 weeks and 15-30% of those between 32 and 36 weeks gestation. It is caused primarily by deficiency of pulmonary surfactant in an immature lung. It can also result from a genetic problem with the production of surfactant associated proteins. RDS is a major cause of morbidity and mortality in preterm infants (4-6). Signs of RDS usually appear within minutes after birth, although they may not be recognised for several hours in larger babies. It results because of an insufficiency of pulmonary surfactant which leads to airway collapse.

It is inefficient for airways and lungs to completely collapse during expiration as re-inflation requires much more energy than widening of a partially closed open airway. Under normal circumstances airway closure is opposed by maintenance of functional residual capacity (FRC) at a level above the point at which airways collapse (the critical closing volume (CCV)). CCV is increased in surfactant deficiency, bronchiolitis and pneumonia. FRC is reduced when lying supine, during anaesthesia and during sleep.

Three factors predominantly influence the FRC: elastic recoil of the chest, the time allowed for expiration and the expiratory flow rate (2). Children will usually attempt to maintain FRC at a level above CCV by several synergistic mechanisms. The newborn child has a limited number of ways to oppose airway closure. Whilst elastic recoil of the chest cannot be varied it does increase with age and hence older children are less susceptible to complete airway closure. Increases in respiratory rate (leading to a shorter expiratory time) and grunting both lead to an increase in FRC. Grunting requires considerable effort itself and is usually a sign of significant illness (1,2). Grunting frequently occurs in combination with nasal flaring and intercostal or subcostal retractions as all three are associated with increased work of breathing. The distinctive sound of grunting is produced when the glottis is closed during expiration. This increases end-expiratory pressure in the lungs (similar to increasing the PEEP setting on a ventilator) and helps to improve oxygenation in children with ventilation perfusion mismatching due to regional airway closure.

As the disease progresses, the baby may develop ventilatory failure and prolonged apnoea. In most cases, the symptoms and signs reach a peak within 3 days, after which improvement is gradual. Improvement is often heralded by spontaneous diuresis.

Surfactant production

Surfactant production begins in the final stage of embryonic lung development (saccular stage (26-36 weeks gestation)). In this stage, formation of alveoli occurs by the outgrowth of septae that subdivide terminal saccules into anatomic alveoli, where air exchange occurs. The number of alveoli in each lung increases from almost zero at 32 week gestation to between 50 and 150 million alveoli in term infants and 300 million in adults. Alveolar growth continues for at least two years after birth at term (2,3,7).

Alveoli are made up of Type I pneumocytes which are essential for gas exchange and Type II pneumocytes which produce surfactant. Surfactant is made of complex system of lipids (accounts for 90% and predominantly disaturated palmitoylphosphatidyl choline), proteins (hydrophobic surfactant proteins SP-B and SP-C and the hydrophilic proteins SP-A and SP-D) and cholesterol.

The surfactant is packaged by the cell in structures called lamellar bodies, and extruded into the air-spaces. The lamellar bodies then unfold into a complex lining of the air-space. This layer reduces the surface tension of the fluid that lines the air-space. Surface tension is responsible for approximately 2/3 of the elastic recoil forces. By reducing surface tension, surfactant prevents the air-spaces from completely collapsing on exhalation. In addition, the decreased surface tension allows re-opening of the air-space with a lower amount of force. Therefore, without adequate amounts of surfactant, the air-spaces collapse and are very difficult to expand.

The major negative effects of surfactant deficiency on pulmonary function are low compliance and low lung volume (functional residual capacity), and are primarily due to atelectasis, although both pulmonary oedema and inflammation may be contributing factors. Total lung resistance is slightly increased, probably as a result of airway compression by interstitial oedema and damage to the airways by the increased pressure needed to expand the poorly compliant alveoli.

Ventilation-perfusion (V/Q) mismatch

Deficient synthesis or release of surfactant, together with small respiratory units and a compliant chest wall produces atelectasis and results in perfused, but not ventilated alveoli (3,7). This causes hypoxia decreased lung compliance, small tidal volumes, increased physiological dead space, increased work of breathing and insufficient alveolar ventilation eventually results in hypercapnia.

Microscopically, a surfactant deficient lung is characterized by collapsed air-spaces alternating with hyper-expanded areas, vascular congestion and in time formation of hyaline membranes (4,7). Hyaline membranes are composed of fibrin, cellular debris, red blood cells, rare neutrophils and macrophages. They appear as an eosinophilic, amorphous material, lining or filling the air spaces and blocking gas exchange.

As a result, blood passing through the lungs is unable to pick up oxygen and unload carbon dioxide. This results in hypoxia, hypercarbia and respiratory acidosis.

Syllabus Mapping

Neonatology

- understand the normal physiological processes occurring during the perinatal period
- understand the physiological basis of neonatal resuscitation
- understand the scientific basis of common diseases and conditions affecting the newborn, including the consequences of prematurity

References

1. RJ, Martin RJ, and Fanaroff, AA. Respiratory distress syndrome and its management. Fanaroff and Martin (eds.) Neonatal-perinatal medicine: Diseases of the fetus and infant; 7th ed. (2002):1001-1011. St. Louis: Mosby.

2. Nelson Textbook of Pediatrics. 19th ed. Philadelphia, Elsevier Saunders; 2011

3. Nkadi PO, Merritt TA, Pillers DA. An overview of pulmonary surfactant in the neonate: genetics, metabolism, and the role of surfactant in health and disease. *Mol Genet Metab* 2009;**97**:95-101.

4. Roberts D, Dalziel S. Antenatal corticosteroids for accelerating fetal lung maturation for women at risk of preterm birth. *Cochrane Database Syst Rev* 2006; CD004454.

5. Schwartz, R.M., Luby, A.M., Scanlon, J.W., & Kellogg, R.J. Effect of surfactant on morbidity, mortality, and resource use in newborn infants weighing 500 to 1500 g. *New Engl J Med* 1994;**330**:1476-1480.

6. Stoll BJ, Hansen NI, Bell EF, et al. Neonatal outcomes of extremely preterm infants from the NICHD Neonatal Research Network. *Pediatrics* 2010;**126**:443-456.

7. Jobe, AH. Lung development and maturation. In: Neonatal-Perinatal Medicine , 2, 9th, Martin RJ, Fanaroff AA, Walsh MC (Eds), Elsevier Mosby, St Louis 2011. p.1075.

Chapter 37: A neonate on a ventilator
Mithila D'Souza

You receive handover from the day team about a 26/40 preterm infant, weighing 1000g, who was born by emergency section due to antepartum haemorrhage. The mother received 1 dose of betamethasone an hour before delivery. The baby was intubated in theatre and given 200mg/Kg of surfactant. The xray shows bilateral ground glass changes. He is settled on 20mcg/Kg/hr of morphine and is currently ventilated on SIMV mode with the current settings.

Ventilatory rate	60 per minute
Inspired oxygen concentration [FiO$_2$]	60%
Positive inspiratory pressure [PIP]	22 cmH$_2$O
Positive end expiratory pressure [PEEP]	6 cmH$_2$O
Inspiratory time [IT]	0.4 seconds
Tidal volume	3.6ml

From the following list of possible ventilator changes (A-J) please select the most appropriate change for each of the following blood gases.

A. Decrease the FiO$_2$
B. Decrease the inspiratory time
C. Decrease the Positive end expiratory pressure (PEEP)
D. Decrease the Positive inspiratory pressure (PIP)
E. Decrease the ventilator rate
F. Increase the FiO$_2$
G. Increase the inspiratory time
H. Increase the PEEP
I. Increase the PIP
J. Increase the ventilator rate

Q1. The neonatal nurse has just done an arterial blood gas which shows:

pH 7.17   pCO$_2$ 8.7 kPa   pO$_2$ 7.6 kPa   HCO$_3$ 23 mmol/L   Base Excess - 4.0

Q2. The neonatal nurse has just done an arterial blood gas which shows:

pH 7.25   pCO$_2$ 6.0 kPa   pO$_2$ 30 kPa   HCO$_3$ 19 mmol/L   Base Excess - 4.0

Q3. The neonatal nurse has just done an arterial blood gas which shows:

pH 7.45   pCO$_2$ 3.6 kPa   pO$_2$ 8.0 kPa   HCO$_3$ 28 mmol/L   Base Excess + 6.0

Answer and Rationale

Q1.   **I. Increase the PIP**
Q2.   **A. Reduce FiO2**
Q3.   **E. Decrease ventilator rate**

Making Ventilator Changes – a very simple users guide

The first thing to determine is whether the baby has a problem with carbon dioxide clearance, oxygenation or both. Your oxygen saturations will give you an indication of how well the baby is oxygenating but must be taken into consideration with the amount of inspired oxygen concentration (FiO_2) required and the arterial oxygen concentration (paO_2). For example, saturations may be 94% but if a FiO_2 of 60% is required to achieve this and the paO_2 generated is only 7.6kPa, there is a problem with oxygenation. On the other hand, the only way to know if a baby is ventilating adequately i.e. clearing carbon dioxide effectively, is by obtaining a blood gas. (See below for refresher on blood gas interpretation).

Initially, when making changes, it is best to think of carbon dioxide clearance and oxygenation separately (although the changes you make, could affect both).

> **CO_2 clearance** is determined by **Minute ventilation** (MV),
> where MV = Tidal Volume (TV) X Respiratory Rate (RR)

> **Oxygenation** is determined by **Mean Airway Pressure** (MAP), where
> $$MAP = \frac{(\text{Inspiratory time (Ti)} \times \text{PIP}) + (\text{Expiratory time (Te)} \times \text{PEEP})}{\text{Inspiratory time (Ti)} + \text{Expiratory time (Te)}}$$

Therefore to **improve oxygenation**

1. **Increase mean airway pressure** by or 2. **Increase FiO₂**

a. Increasing PEEP
b. Increasing PIP
c. Increasing inspiration time

Figure 37.1. *Generation of the mean airway pressure*

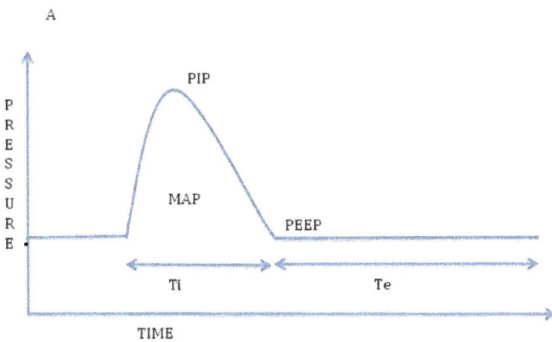

As we spend a greater time in expiration, increasing the PEEP will give the greatest increase in the area under the curve and therefore have the greatest affect on MAP. However, remember that increasing PEEP will also reduce tidal volume and subsequently reduce carbon dioxide (CO_2) clearance. Additionally, there is a limit to how high we can increase PEEP, as eventually the alveoli will become over distended, impeding alveolar capillary blood flow and leading to ventilation perfusion mismatch.

Increasing your PIP will have a greater affect on MAP, than increasing the inspiratory time.   Increasing PIP will also cause an increase in tidal volume and improve carbon dioxide clearance, which may be favourable.

Increasing inspiratory time may be more useful in situations where the PIP is already very high. Longer inspiratory time will also allow sufficient time for the high pressures to be achieved therefore opening the stiff lungs more gently. Be mindful that by increasing inspiratory time, at a set rate, you are then reducing the time for expiration, which will also influence the baby's ability to clear carbon dioxide. If the inspiratory time is longer than the expiratory time the patient will start to air trap and develop auto PEEP, leading to over distension of alveoli and increasing the risk of pneumothorax or pulmonary interstitial emphysema.

Weaning Ventilation

Generally if your pH is normal, you may be able to make a change even if the CO_2 is above normal limits (permissive hypercapnia) and especially if the CO_2 is low as this will affect cerebral perfusion. You must also predict what effect your changes will make. If the pH is borderline, like in question 2, any changes that decrease CO_2 clearance may result in acidosis. Deciding on whether you change your PIP, tidal volume or rate will depend on what tidal volumes are being generated, how high your PIP is and how much the baby is breathing for themselves, but the overall aim is to avoid lung trauma from unnecessary pressures and volumes. However, if oxygenation is still a problem, it may not be possible for you to alter variables that will have a significant affect on MAP. Most people will only make changes affecting oxygenation when FiO_2 is down to at least 40%, unless significant pressures are being used, then it is beneficial to reduce these earlier if possible.

Table 37.1: Refresher of Blood gas interpretation

	Parameters	Normal	Acidosis	Alkalosis
1. Acid or Alkali?	pH	7.25 – 7.35	<7.25	>7.35
2. Respiratory cause?	CO_2	4.6 - 6		-
3. Metabolic cause?	HCO_3 BE	22-26 -2 to +2	-	

pH	CO2	HCO3	Interpretation
Normal	Normal	Normal	Normal
< 7.25		Normal	Respiratory acidosis
<7.25	Normal	-	Metabolic acidosis
<7.25		-	Mixed Resp & Metabolic acidosis
Normal			Compensated Resp acidosis
Normal	-	-	Compensated Metabolic acidosis
>7.35	-	Normal	Respiratory Alkalosis
>7.35	Normal		Metabolic Alkalosis
>7.35	-		Mixed Resp & Metabolic alkalosis

Syllabus Mapping

Neonatology

• understand the principles of mechanical ventilation including the interpretation of blood gases

References and Further Reading

1. Workbook in Practical Neonatology 4th Edition. Polin RA & Yoder AR 2007.

2. Fetal & Neonatal Secrets 2nd Edition. Polin RA & Spitzer AR 2006.

Chapter 38: A preterm infant with hyponatraemia Dr Lisa Barker

On the neonatal unit ward round you see a male infant, just under 1 day old, born at 32+6 weeks gestation by emergency cesarean section due to fetal distress. Two doses of antenatal steroids were given prior to delivery. He was born in poor condition and required noninvasive ventilation for 3 minutes. APGAR scores were 6 at 1 minute and 9 at 5 minutes. Cord blood sampling showed a pH of 7.20 and a base excess of -10.8. This is mum's second pregnancy. She previously had a son that died at 6 months of age.

He is in an incubator receiving 28% oxygen. He is receiving intravenous fluid via a cannula and has started minimal enteral feeds of expressed breast milk via a nasogastric tube, which he is tolerating well. On examination he is mildly jaundiced, he has mild subcostal recession. He has normal heart sounds and palpable femoral pulses.

His urine output is currently 2.3mls/Kg/hr. He had bloods taken this morning, the electrolytes are as follows: Sodium 129mmol/L, Potassium 4.5 mmol/L, Urea 5.4 mmol/L, Creatinine 72 µmol/L.

Q1. What is the most likely cause of the hyponatraemia?

A. Increased natriuresis due to prematurity
B. Maternal intravenous fluid prior to delivery
C. Transepidermal fluid loss
D. Respiratory distress syndrome
E. Perinatal asphyxia

Q2. You are asked to prescribe a new bag of fluid. What fluid would you prescribe?

A. 10% glucose
B. 10% glucose with 3mmol/Kg/day sodium chloride
C. 10% glucose with 3mmol/Kg/day sodium chloride and 2mmol/Kg/day potassium
D. 10% glucose with 2mmol/Kg/day potassium chloride
E. Stop the intravenous fluid

Answers and Rationale

Q1.   B. Maternal intravenous fluids prior to delivery

Q2.   A. 10% glucose

This question looks at factors affecting sodium and water balance in the newborn infant and requires an understanding of physiological processes unique to the preterm infant. Fluid management in the preterm infant is critical in preventing morbidity and mortality (1).

Very early on in life (within the first 24 hours), sodium balance is affected by maternal sodium balance. Maternal hyponatraemia can occur as a consequence of; large amounts of rapidly given fluid as may occur in resuscitation for hypotension, glucose only intravenous fluid infusions and the use of oxytocin. All of which may occur during an emergency instrumental delivery. Most amniotic fluid is derived from maternal tissue (interstitial fluid) by diffusion across the amniochorionic membrane. The water content of the amniotic fluid changes every 3 hours (2). Rapid movement of sodium occurs across the placenta so that maternal and fetal sodium is in balance (3), thus maternal hyponatraemia will give rise to fetal hyponatraemia. The hyponatraemia will resolve as extracellular fluid is lost during the diuresis that occurs in all infants, term and preterm. Extracellular fluid loss occurs through a postnatal diuresis that happens in the first 2 or 3 days of life and causes a 10-15% weight loss seen in all infants during the first week of life (4,5). While hyponatraemia in the newborn infant within the first 24 hours of life may be dismissed as just reflecting maternal sodium level, a significant hyponatraemia in the newborn infant should be discussed with healthcare professionals involved in the care of the mother and acted upon as necessary.

Premature and low/extremely low birth weight infants experience disproportionately large insensible fluid losses. This is due to their relatively large body surface area and immature skin. Transepidermal water loss from the interstitial space results in a hyperosmolar extracellular space and thus hypernatraemia, not hyponatraemia, would be observed. Massive insensible transepidermal water loss can occur in preterm infants nursed under radiant heaters. With the use of humidified incubators, transepidermal water loss and hypernatraemia is reduced, but can still occur if humidification is not managed carefully (5).

Preterm infants with respiratory distress syndrome have a delay in the usual postnatal diuresis. Clinically, we may observe a period of reduced urine output (<2mls/Kg/hr) and as a consequence oedema and a 'dilutional' hyponatraemia due to excess water. This picture can be exacerbated if excess intravenous fluid is given and if this does occur, the fluid volume should be reduced rather than adding sodium to the fluid. An improvement in respiratory status is often seen with the onset of an increased urine output indicating the onset of postnatal diuresis. The onset of this fluid loss is determined by cardiopulmonary adaptation and not renal maturation as is often thought (5). Antenatal steroid treatment and postnatal surfactant can improve respiratory status and this classical picture may not be as clinically obvious.

Perinatal asphyxia where severe hypoxia or hypotension is present can result in acute renal failure, with a period or oliguria or anuria, and can also bring on syndrome of inappropriate antidiuretic hormone (SIADH). The infant in the case described above does not fit with a picture of perinatal asphyxia.

Preterm infants have an increased natriuresis (sodium loss in urine) due to prematurity. Infants after 32-33 weeks gestation are able to produce virtually sodium-free urine (4). This commonly leads to the development of hyponatraemia by the second or third week of life in preterm infants if intake is inadequate. Extremely premature infants born before 28 weeks gestation can have very large renal losses of up to 10mmol/Kg/day (5) and this can result in hyponatraemia after the first few days of life. In newborn infants the proximal tubule of the kidney absorbs a smaller fraction of sodium resulting in increased delivery to the distal tubule. In extremely preterm infants, due to immaturity, the distal tubule cannot compensate and the result is natriuresis, negative salt balance and hyponatraemia (4).

Sodium supplementation should be given after the first 24-48 hours, after some weight loss has been seen (5). Intravenous fluids or parenteral nutrition are often required for the preterm infant while enteral feeds are established. Due to the physiological changes discussed above, it is not appropriate to give additional sodium in the first 24-48 hours of life. Many neonatal units have their own guidance for starting and increasing intravenous fluids. Before changes are made to the fluid (volume or content) a full assessment of fluid balance including weight, urine output, volumes in and volumes out and recent electrolytes should be made.

Syllabus Mapping

Neonatology

- understand the normal physiological processes occurring during the perinatal period
- understand the principles of fluid and electrolyte management and nutrition in the neonate.

Pharmacology, poisoning and accidents

- understand the mode of action, physiological and metabolic mechanisms of therapeutic agents, including intravenous fluids

References

1. Bhatia J. Fluid and electrolyte management in the very low birth weight neonate. *J Perinatol* 2006;**26 suppl 1**:S19-21.

2. Moore KL, Persaud TVN. Placenta and fetal membranes. In. Before we are born. Essentials of Enbryology and Birth Defects (5th Edition). Saunders 1998:139-142.

3. Roberts TJ, Nijland MJM, Williams L, Ross MG. Fetal diuretic response to maternal hyponatraemia:contribution of placental sodium gradient. *J Appl Physiol* 1999;**87**:1440-1447.

4. Haycock G. Renal Function and renal disease in the newborn. Disorders of the kidney and urinary tract. In:Roberton's Textbook of Neonataology. Fourth Edition. Elsevier Churchill Livingstone 2005: 932-934.

5. Modi N. Management of fluid balance in the very immature neonate. *Arch Dis Child Fetal Neonatal Ed* 2004;**89**:F108-111.

Chapter 39: A diuresis in a teenager with a head injury Dr Patrick Davies

A 14 year old boy is admitted to the emergency department after a road traffic accident. He was cycling without a helmet, and was hit by a car travelling at 30 mph. At the scene he had a Glasgow Coma Score of 5. He was intubated at the road side and taken to hospital. On arrival he had a CT scan of the head which showed a large left parietal skull fracture, a thin extra axial haemorrhage, and an element of swelling over both hemispheres. No other injuries were found on full examination.

He was transferred to the paediatric intensive care unit, and the neurosurgeons inserted an intracranial bolt for pressure monitoring. At 36 hours, his intracranial pressure was at a baseline of 20 cmH$_2$0, with spikes up to 30 cmH$_2$0. His urine output begins to rise, and his serum sodium is falling.

Q1.   Which of the following conditions are most likely?

A.   Central diabetes insipidus
B.   Cerebral salt wasting
C.   Exogenous excess fluids during resuscitation
D.   Hyponatraemic dehydration
E.   Syndrome of inappropriate anti diuretic hormone (SIADH)

Q2.   What is the best treatment for this child?

A.   Decrease fluid amount, decrease sodium load
B.   Decrease fluid amount, increase sodium load
C.   Increase fluid amount, decrease sodium load
D.   Increase fluid amount, increase sodium load
E.   Leave things as they are: this is a physiological response

Answers and Rationale

Q1.   **B. Cerebral salt wasting**

Q2.   **D. Increase fluid amount, increase sodium load**

Fluid management in children with head injury can be complex, confusing, and needs a good understanding of the physiological mechanisms behind the effects seen. As always, the more data which can be put in to the puzzle, the easier it becomes to come to an answer.

The first question to pose is this: is the kidney working properly and normally? Is the kidney trying to respond properly, and responding to the stimuli it is getting (either physically, or hormonally)? If the kidney is damaged, which in trauma patients can be by physical trauma, or by secondary effects, for instance a period of severe hypotension or hypoxia at the roadside, then everything changes. The answers and rationale in this case presumes a normal kidney. Any properly worded question will address this.

There are five distinct problems these children can develop. In "real life", some children get combinations of 2 or even 3 of these, which makes things extraordinarily complex, but for the purposes of exams you would be handed a patient who fits in to one category.

Exogenous excess fluids during resuscitation

This is a real risk, especially in teenagers who are treated by adult doctors as if they are adults. Fortunately, hypotonic fluids are now not used for resuscitation, which makes the potential for fluid shifts much less. However, children who are over-resuscitated will, presuming a normal kidney, develop a large diuresis, and on occasion may "overshoot". This would give a picture of high urine output hyponatraemia, but this would happen early in the illness. The case, as given, is of a late development of this problem. It is also more likely that they will become hypernatraemic, due to excess sodium given in normal saline resuscitation, which overloads the body sodium stores. High serum sodium however is welcomed in patients with raised ICP as it helps to reduce intracranial pressure.

There are four further causes. More clinical and biochemical data will aid decision making.

Syndrome of Inappropriate Anti Diuretic Hormone (SIADH)

Patients with SIADH are fluid overloaded. They have an excess of anti diuretic hormone (also called vasopressin), which is a nine amino acid hormone secreted from the posterior pituitary. It has an effect on the collecting ducts of the kidney, and promotes the reabsorbtion of water from the tubules back in to the blood. The collecting ducts, within the medulla of the kidney, are bathed in fluid with an osmolality of between 600-1200 mosm/L. ADH alters the permeability in this region, so the more ADH which is available, the more permeable the membrane becomes, and therefore the more water is drawn out of the tubules. At the distal convoluted tubule 7% of the glomerular filtrate is still within the nephron, and this can drop to as little as 0.5%. This is the most common sodium balance problem in post head injury cases: and the causes for this are not yet properly understood. Patients will have a low urine output. They are conserving fluid (inappropriately), despite their relatively high intravascular filling. The urine which is passed will be very concentrated, both for osmolality and sodium. Treatment for these patients is fluid restriction, despite their low urine output. There will be a gradual resolution.

Dehydration

Dehydration can manifest itself as normo-, hypo-, or hypernatraemic, depending on the relative amounts of fluid and sodium which have been lost. However, these will be patients with low amounts of urine, and high serum and urine osmolalities. They try to preserve their sodium (as they have lost body sodium during their dehydrating illness), so urine sodium will be low. Treatment is by rehydration. As a rule, rehydration at the pace at which the dehydration occurred should keep the patient safe. Too rapid rehydration can cause fluid shifts which can be dangerous. Rapid increases of sodium can cause central pontine myelinolysis, a permanent brain damage. Always start with normal saline, monitor frequently, then change as needed.

Central Diabetes Insipidus

Central DI is the opposite of SIADH: in this case there is not enough ADH available. This is usually caused by a direct dysfunction of the posterior pituitary, disrupting the normal supply of the hormone. Without ADH, much more, dilute urine is produced. This is a complication seen in severe head injuries. In central DI the problem is one of water loss: therefore the body becomes dehydrated, but whilst producing a high urine output. Serum osmolality is high, but urine osmolality is low, with a low urinary sodium. Treatment is with the synthetic ADH analogue, Desmopressin. The effect of treatment is dramatic and often almost instantaneous.

Cerebral salt wasting

Cerebral salt wasting is a rare but important complication of head injuries. The cause for this is unclear, but seems to be due to an abnormality of the proximal tubule of the nephron, where excess sodium is lost. This then draws water with it, leading to a hyponatraemic dehydration state. One possible cause is that sympathetic overdrive in head injury, causes local hypertension and that the kidney's response is simply a 'normal' hypertension-natriuresis response. The biochemical picture is mixed, with a high urea, but low serum osmolality and high urinary sodium. Treatment is by replacing fluid to ensure euvolaemia, and replacing sodium to balance the urinary losses.

Investigations necessary

Urinary electrolytes are a critical part of the analysis of fluid and electrolyte balances. Without a knowledge of what is lost, it becomes very difficult to understand the process which has resulted in blood electrolyte disturbances. The table below is a summary of the changes which are seen in the different conditions.

	SIADH	CSW	DI	Dehydration
Serum sodium	Low (<135)	Low (<135)	High (>145)	Low / normal / high
Serum urea	Low / normal	High	High	High
Serum osmolality	Low (<275)	Low (<275)	High (>300)	High
CVP	High (>8)	Low (<4)	Low (<4)	Low (<4)
Urine output	Low	High	High (>4 ml/Kg/hr)	Low
Urine specific gravity	High (>1010)	Normal / high (>1010)	Low (<1010)	High
U Osm	High	Normal / high	Low	High
Urine osmolality	High (>20)	Very High(10 x N)	Low (<20)	Low (< 20)
Urine osmaolality/ Serum osmolality	High (>1.5)	High (>1)	Low (<1)	
Treatment	**Fluid restriction**	**Replace fluid and replace sodium**	**Desmopressin**	**Replace fluid**

Syllabus Mapping

Neurology and neurodisability

- understand the physiological and pathophysiological changes that occur in neurological disorders, including migraine, raised intracranial pressure, idiopathic intracranial hypertension, epilepsy

Nephro-urology

- understand the disease associations of renal conditions with other conditions

References and Further Reading

1. Despopoulos, A., & Silbernagl, S. *Color atlas of physiology.* 2003. George Thieme Verlag.

Acknowledgements

Electrolyte table courtesy of Professor Harish Vyas, Nottingham University.

Chapter 40: The mode of action of diuretics
Dr Jo Campion-Smith

A 4 month old baby known to have a ventriculoseptal defect is admitted with a history of poor feeding, faltering growth and signs of respiratory distress. You note that he has been on regular furosemide for the last 6 weeks. After a full clinical assessment, baseline bloods and a gas are done.

Q1. Considering the mechanism of action of furosemide, which pattern of results would be most likely?

A.   Hyperkalaemia, hyponatraemia, hyperchloraemia, metabolic alkalosis
B.   Hyperkalaemia, hyponatraemia, hypochloraemia, metabolic alkalosis
C.   Hypokalaemia, hypernatraemia, hypochloraemia, metabolic acidosis
D.   Hypokalaemia, hyponatraemia, hypochloraemia, metabolic acidosis
E.   Hypokalaemia, hyponatraemia, hypochloraemia, metabolic alkalosis

A 14 year old child was admitted the previous evening with confusion and diabetic ketoacidosis. The on call medical team treated her with mannitol. This morning she is alert and cooperative but clinically remains dehydrated.

Q2. In this context, how does mannitol exacerbate dehydration?

A.   Mannitol acts on the proximal convoluted tubule to increase sodium and thus water excretion
B.   Mannitol antagonises the action of aldosterone in the distal convoluted tubule and collecting ducts
C.   Mannitol binds to the aquaporin-2 receptor in the collecting ducts, reducing permeability to water
D.   Mannitol blocks the Na^+-K^+-2Cl co-transporter thus increasing sodium and water excretion
E.   Mannitol is freely filtered at Bowman's capsule, increasing tubular osmolality and thus water excretion

Answers and Rationale

Q1.   E. Hypokalaemia, hyponatraemia, hypochloraemia, metabolic alkalosis

Q2.   E. Mannitol is freely filtered at Bowman's capsule, increasing tubular osmolality and thus water excretion

In order to answer these questions reliably, it is necessary to understand renal tubular function, the hormones which influence renal function and the site and mechanism of action of diuretics.

Renal tubular function – a brief review

The nephron is the basic functional unit of the kidney and it is here that the processes of ultrafiltration, reabsorption and secretion of electrolytes and water occur in order to generate urine. The nephron's structure reflects its function which is summarised as follows:

The nephron begins at the Bowman's capsule where ultrafiltration of blood at the glomerular capillary wall occurs. Ultrafiltration is a passive process which is dependent on 3 factors: renal blood flow, the oncotic pressure of plasma and hydrostatic pressure. The high pressure pushes small molecules (organic solutes and inorganic ions) through the glomerular capillary wall into Bowman's capsule. Large, negatively charged ions, such as proteins, are repelled by the negative charge of the glomerular basement membrane. Thus no blood or platelets and virtually no protein are filtered. The ultrafiltrate then passes into the proximal convoluted tubule (PCT). Up to 99% of filtered sodium is reabsorbed in the renal tubule (1). Of this, approximately two thirds is actively reabsorbed in the PCT (1) by the Na^+/K^+ ATPase pump. Also reabsorbed in the PCT are amino acids, chloride, glucose, phosphate, urea, bicarbonate, calcium and potassium (2, 3). A secondary method of sodium reabsorption is through coupling with these substrates. The solute reabsorption within the PCT creates an osmotic gradient prompting 70% of filtered water to be reabsorbed. From the PCT, filtrate moves into the Loop of Henle. 25% of filtered sodium is reabsorbed, by the $Na^+K^+2Cl^-$ co-transporter. Pooling of sodium chloride in the medullary interstitium generates a concentration gradient which enables concentration of urine (countercurrent multiplication). The most concentrated part of the medullary interstitium is around the tip of the loops of Henle and this concentration affects water reabsorption from the collecting ducts. On arrival in the distal convoluted tubule (DCT), the filtrate is now hypotonic. The DCT walls are impermeable to water but contain a pump which reabsorbs approximately 5% of filtered sodium in exchange for potassium or hydrogen. This pump is controlled by aldosterone. Finally the urine passes through the collecting ducts, which pass close to the tips of the loops of Henle. Water diffuses passively out of the collecting duct depending on the permeability of the duct and the concentration gradient in the medullary interstitium at the tip of the loop of Henle. Urine concentration is determined by antidiuretic hormone, which acts on the aquaporin-2 water channel, increasing the permeability of the ducts to water, facilitating water uptake and thus concentrating the urine. A further 2% of sodium can be reabsorbed in exchange for potassium, which again is controlled by aldosterone.

Hormonal control of renal function

Antidiuretic hormone (ADH) determines urine concentration and volume by increasing collecting duct permeability and thus water reabsorption. ADH is released by the posterior pituitary in response to increased plasma osmolality.

Reduced renal perfusion and low sodium levels in the distal tubule cause renin release, which converts angiotensinogen to angiotensin I. Angiotensin I is converted to angiotensin II by the angiotensin converting enzyme, which in turn causes vasoconstriction and an increased release of aldosterone. Aldosterone acts in the DCT and collecting ducts to promote sodium and water reabsorption (in exchange for hydrogen and potassium), which increases the circulating volume. As well as being stimulated by angiotensin II, it is also synthesised in response to raised extracellular potassium levels. A-type and B-type natriuretic peptides are hormones which have both central and peripheral effects. With respect to renal function, they antagonise the renin-angiotensin-aldosterone pathway (4) and cause vasodilation and increased sodium and water excretion (2).

Diuretics

Diuretics are agents which promote water and electrolyte excretion and are predominantly used in conditions of fluid overload, electrolyte imbalance and renal failure. They are classified according to their mechanism of action and it is this which determines their specific clinical indications and their impact on plasma biochemistry.

Loop diuretics – e.g. furosemide. As suggested by their name, loop diuretics act in the loop of Henle where they block the $Na^+K^+2Cl^-$ co-transporter. In doing so, there is increased excretion of sodium, chloride and potassium as well as water (due to a reduced concentration gradient in the medullary interstitium at the tip of the loop of Henle). Use of loop diuretics can lead to hypovolaemia, hyponatraemia, hypokalaemia and hypochloraemia. In response to low potassium there is reabsorption of potassium with secretion of hydrogen, resulting in a metabolic alkalosis (5). This reabsorption of potassium is not enough to prevent hypokalaemia. Increased excretion of calcium (leading to hypercalciuria) and magnesium (causing hypomagnesaemia) also occurs (1).

Thiazide diuretics – e.g. chlorthiazide. Thiazide diuretics act in the DCT by inhibiting sodium chloride reabsorption. Only 5% of sodium is reabsorbed in the DCT and thus there is only a small increase in the overall amount of sodium chloride excreted and their diuretic effect is relatively weak. Side effects include hyponatraemia, hypokalaemia and a metabolic alkalosis. Thiazide diuretics also increase the reabsorption of calcium in the DCT and can therefore cause hypercalcaemia (1). Chronic diuretic therapy (both loop and thiazide diuretics) also causes hyperuricaemia by increasing reabsorption of uric acid in the proximal tubule, secondary to volume depletion, and as the diuretic itself competes for secretion in the proximal tubule with uric acid, thereby reducing the amount of uric acid secreted (6).

Aldosterone-antagonists – e.g. spironolactone. By blocking the action of aldosterone in the DCT and collecting ducts, sodium and water excretion is increased. However, in contrast to other diuretics, potassium and hydrogen are 'spared' as they are no longer secreted in exchange for sodium. Thus side effects include hyperkalaemia and a metabolic acidosis.

Osmotic diuretics – e.g. mannitol. Osmotic diuretics act by altering the osmotic pressure in the renal tubule. They are freely filtered at Bowman's capsule and increase the osmolality of the filtrate within the tubule which reduces water (and subsequently sodium chloride) reabsorption. Excretion of all electrolytes is increased (1). For further details concerning the mechanisms of action of mannitol see chapter 34.

Syllabus Mapping

Nephro-urology
- understand the physiology of normal kidney and bladder
- understand the pharmacology of agents commonly used in renal disorders

Cardiology
- understand the pharmacology of drugs used to treat common cardiac conditions, including duct dependant cyanosis, heart failure and arrhythmias

Pharmacology, poisoning and accidents
- understand the mode of action, physiological and metabolic mechanisms of therapeutic agents, including intravenous fluids
- understand the planned undesired effects of therapeutic agents
- understand the pharmacokinetics of commonly used medicines and the relationship to renal and other organ function

References

1. Gaon P. (2000). *Paediatric Exams - A Survival Guide.* Elsevier Churchill Livingstone, 67-68.

2. Guignard J.P. (2006). Diuretics. In; Jacqz-Aigrain E. & Choonara I. (eds), *Paediatric Clinical Pharmacology*. Lausanne, New York; FontisMedia and Taylor & Francis, 737-753.

3. Kliegman R.M. & Stanton B. F. et al. (2011). Nelson Textbook of Pediatrics. 19th ed. Philadelphia, Elsevier Saunders; 2011. pp235-6 & online content

4. Spieker LE, *et al.* The management of hyperuricemia and gout in patients with heart failure. *Eur J Heart Failure* 2002;**4**:403-410.

5. Gardiner M, Eisen S, & Murphy C. (2009), *Training in Paediatrics – the Essential Curriculum.* Oxford University Press, 120-121, 432.

6. Suzuki T, Yamazaki T, Yazaki Y. The role of the natriuretic peptides in the cardiovascular system. *Cardiovasc Research* 2001;**51**:489-494.

Acknowledgements

The author and editor would like to thank Dr. Ian Petransky, Paediatric Registrar & Medical Educator, Royal Derby Hospital, for his assistance reviewing this chapter.

Chapter 41: The child with kidney and lung problems Dr Nicholas Ware

Case 1

A 7 year old boy presents to the emergency department with a three day history of worsening lethargy, dark urine and oliguria. His BP is 128/91mmHg and his urine dipstick shows mild proteinuria. On taking a further history it becomes apparent that he had a throat infection two weeks ago requiring antibiotic treatment from his GP.

Q1. Which was the most likely cause of his throat infection?

A.   Adenovirus
B.   Epstein Barr virus
C.   Group A Streptococcus
D.   Mycoplasma pneumoniae
E.   Staphylococcus aureus

Q2. Given the most likely underlying diagnosis are the following statements true or false?

A.   ASOT is likely to be raised
B.   C4 is usually low
C.   Furosemide will usually lower blood pressure in this context
D.   Renal biopsy is indicated if proteinuria persists at 4 months
E.   Treatment with penicillin will help reduce the proteinuria

Case 2

Later that day a 10 year old girl presents with similar symptoms of worsening lethargy, reduced urine output and dark urine. She reports feeling unwell for over a week and has come to the emergency department due to an episode of haemoptysis. She is admitted and seen by the renal team who think Goodpasture's syndrome is the most likely diagnosis.

Q3. Which ONE of the following blood test results would confirm their suspicion?

A.   Low C3
B.   Presence of anti-glomerular basement membrane (anti-GBM) antibodies
C.   Presence of anti-Ro antibodies
D.   Presence of double-stranded DNA (dsDNA)
E.   Raised antinuclear antibodies (ANA)

Answers and Rationale

Q1. C. Group A Streptococcus
Q2. A. True   B. False   C. True   D. False   E. False
Q3. B. Presence of anti-glomerular basement membrane (anti-GBM) antibodies

The symptoms and signs described in both case 1 and case 2 are typical of acute nephritis. Acute nephritis is a glomerular injury that presents as acute kidney failure (oliguria, uraemia and elevated creatinine) typically combined with hypertension, haematuria, oedema and proteinuria. The hypertension is due to salt and water retention and hence often responds to treatment with the loop diuretic furosemide [see chapter 40]. Haematuria can be microscopic or macroscopic and red cell casts are seen on urine microscopy. Proteinuria can reach nephrotic range (>200mg/mmol) although is usually not this high. It is therefore important that any patient presenting with symptoms or signs of acute kidney injury have a urine dipstick and have their BP checked, ideally using a manual sphygmomanometer. It is also important to do a renal ultrasound scan. In cases of nephritis the ultrasound scan will usually be normal but is necessary to exclude other causes of haematuria and reduced renal function.

In case 1 the recent sore throat makes a post-infectious cause of nephritis most likely. The commonest causative organism is group A beta-haemolytic Streptococcus and the onset of symptoms is typically 1-2 weeks after a throat infection or up to 6 weeks after a skin infection. Antistreptolysin O titre (ASOT) is raised in the majority of throat infections although not after many skin infections. Remember that it is also positive in up to 20% of healthy children and so must be interpreted with caution.

In addition to group A beta-haemolytic Streptococcus there are a number of other organisms that can cause post-infectious glomerulonephritis. These include bacteria such as Staphylococcus aureus, Escherichia coli, Streptococcus pneumonia, Mycoplasma pneumonia, Campylobacter, Salmonella and tuberculosis, as well as certain viruses (such as Epstein-Barr virus, cytomegalovirus, herpes simplex virus, varicella-zoster virus and hepatitis B/C), fungi (such as Candida, Aspergillus and histoplasmosis) and parasites (such as malaria, toxoplasmosis and schistosomiasis).

It is known that post-infectious nephritis is caused by an immunological process although the exact mechanism is still not certain. The most supported theory is that of immune-complex mediated glomerular damage whereby antigenic determinants are formed with a direct affinity for sites within the glomerulus. In addition glomerular bound antibodies serve as fixed antigens and immune complexes form leading to complement fixation. This then triggers the classical complement pathway leading to the production of additional inflammatory mediators and recruitment of inflammatory cells which leads to glomerular damage.

In post-streptococcal glomerulonephritis treatment with penicillin is necessary to prevent spread to contacts but does not alter the nephritis, the severity of which is variable but which typically resolves within 2-3 weeks. C3 is usually low while C4 is usually normal (unlike in membranoproliferative glomerulonephritis (MPGN), SLE and endocarditis). C3 returns to normal by 6-8 weeks. Renal biopsy is not indicated unless either the creatinine remains abnormal at 6 weeks, the low C3 persists beyond 3 months or the proteinuria persists beyond 6 months. Microscopic haematuria can sometimes persist for 1-2 years however is not of long term clinical significance. The long term prognosis for children with post-infectious GN is excellent with only 1% going on to develop chronic kidney disease.

Goodpasture's syndrome is rare in children but is important to consider in 'pulmonary-renal syndromes' characterised by nephritis and pulmonary haemorrhage (usually alveolar haemorrhage). Other causes of pulmonary-renal syndromes include SLE, Wegener's granulomatosis, microscopic polyangitis and HSP. Goodpasture's syndrome is also an autoimmune immune complex mediated disease and apart from lungs and kidneys there is usually no other system involvement. The presence of anti-glomerular basement membrane (anti-GBM) antibodies in blood confirms the diagnosis. It is important that treatment is started early and this is usually a combination of corticosteroids and cyclophosphamide as well as plasmapheresis. (Note that anti-GBM antibodies sometimes also form following renal transplantation for Alport's syndrome).

Children with Goodpasture's syndrome need to be referred to a specialist renal unit promptly as there is good evidence that early treatment improves prognosis. Children under the age of five have poorer outcomes and are more likely to progress to chronic kidney disease than older children.

Syllabus Mapping

Nephro-urology

* understand the pathophysiology and the histopathological changes that occur in renal disorders
* understand the pathophysiological mechanisms resulting in hypertension
* understand the pharmacology of agents commonly used in renal disorders
* understand the disease associations of renal conditions with other conditions e.g. HUS, deafness, hepatorenal syndrome

References and Further Reading

1. Rees L et al. (2012). *Paediatric Nephrology.* Oxford University Press.

2. Khanna R. Clinical presentation & management of glomerular diseases: hematuria, nephritic and nephrotic syndrome. *Molecular medicine* 2011;**108(1)**:33-6.

3. Bayat A et al. Characteristics and outcome of Goodpasture's disease in children. *Clinical Rheumatology* 2012;**31(12)**:1745-51.

Chapter 42: Pharmacology of antiepileptic drugs Dr Elizabeth Starkey

Here is a list of mechanisms of actions for anticonvulsants

A.   Calcium channel blocker
B.   Carbonic anhydrase inhibitor
C.   GABA transaminase inhibitor
D.   GABA reuptake inhibitor
E.   GABA receptors agonist
F.   Glutamate receptor antagonist
G.   Multiple mechanisms of action
H.   Potassium channel opener
I.   SV2A-binding agent
J.   Voltage gated sodium channels blocker

Choose the most appropriate mechanism of action for the each of the anti epileptic used in the following scenarios.

SELECT ONE ANSWER ONLY FOR EACH QUESTION

Note: Each answer may be used more than once

Q1.   A 5 year old boy admitted to the children's emergency department with prolonged generalised tonic clonic seizure requiring a dose of buccal midazolam.

Q2.   A 7 year old girl was referred with a history of vacant episodes at school and home affecting her academic work. Hyperventilation in clinic precipitated an absence seizure. She was started on ethosuximide.

Q3.   A 9 month old was admitted to the children's ward with short lived flexion movements in both arms. An EEG showed hypsarrhythmia. Clinical examination revealed ash leaf macules in her groin. She was commenced on vigabatrin.

Answers and Rationale

Q1. **E. GABA receptor agonist**
Q2. **A. Calcium channel blocker**
Q3. **C. GABA transaminase inhibitor**

Understanding the mechanism of action of the antiepileptic drugs (AEDs) is important to enable rational treatment decisions. AEDs work by either decreasing neuronal excitation or enhancing neuronal inhibition by various mechanisms. Different seizure types respond differentially to medicines as they have different underlying causes. If a medicine from one group is effective but not tolerated then a medicine from the same group may be indicated. Similarly, a child who does not benefit from a particular agent will be somewhat less likely to benefit from a drug with a similar mechanism of action. The known mechanisms of action of some of the commoner AEDs are summarised below.

Drug	Voltage gated Na channel	Voltage gated Ca channel	GABA receptor	GABA turnover	Glutamate receptor blocker	Carbonic anhydrase inhibitor	SVA2 binder
Phenobarbitone		+	+++		+		
Phenytoin	+++						
Sodium Valproate	++	++		++			
Carbamazepine	+++						
Benzodiazepine			+++				
Ethosuximide		+++					
Lamotrigine	+++	++					
Topiramate	++	++	++		++	+	
Vigabatrin				+++			
Levetiracetam		+	+				+++
Gabapentin	+	++		+			

(+ + + = principal target, + + = probable target, + = possible target)

Gamma-aminobutyric acid (GABA) is an inhibitory neurotransmitter that is widely distributed throughout the central nervous system. The ubiquitous nature of GABA ensures that any agent increasing GABA activity will tend to reduce seizure frequency and these agents are helpful in treatment of a wide range of seizure types. Benzodiazepines and barbiturates act directly on subunits of the post synaptic GABA receptor-chloride channel complex. Barbiturates increase the duration of chloride channel openings, while benzodiazepines increase the frequency of these openings.

Vigabatrin and tiagabine alter the cellular disposition of GABA. Tiagabine inhibits GABA re-uptake from synapses whereas vigabatrin elevates GABA levels by irreversibly inhibiting GABA-transaminase enzyme (GABA-T). Other antiepileptic agents, including sodium valproate, gabapentin and topiramate have also been reported to influence GABA turnover by increasing neurotransmitter synthesis and/or release.

Sodium valproate is a good example of an AED with known multiple mechanisms of action. Along with lamotrigine and topirimate it has mixed and incompletely understood mechanisms of action.

A number of AEDs act on voltage-gated calcium channels. These channels contribute to the overall electrical excitability of neurones. They are closely involved in neuronal burst firing, and are responsible for the control of neurotransmitter release at pre-synaptic nerve terminals. Ethosuximide exerts its anti-absence effects by blocking T-type calcium voltage-gate currents in thalamocortical relay neurones. The low threshold T-type calcium channel predominates in these neurones where it is believed to play a fundamental role in generating the characteristic 3-Hz spike-and-wave discharge of absence epilepsy. Ethosuximide blocks T-type calcium channels and prevents the synchronised firing. Sodium valproate may have a similar action and may explain why it can also be useful in the treatment of absence seizures. Other AEDS also work on calcium channels including lamotrigine and levetiracetam.

AEDS that affect voltage dependent sodium channels prevent the return of the channels to their active state by stabilizing their inactive form. Sodium channel-blocking AEDs such as phenytoin and carbamazepine bind to the active state of the channel and reduce high frequency firing which occurs during a seizure but allow normal action potentials to occur. Newer AEDs such as lamotrigine and topiramate act by facilitating the fast inactivation of sodium channels. AEDS that affect sodium channels are generally effective treatment for both localised and generalised epilepsy.

Glutamate is one of the most important excitatory neurotransmitters in the brain. Following release it exerts effects on certain receptors in the postsynaptic membrane and this glutamate binding results in neuronal excitation. No AEDS specifically target these glutamate receptors however several newer treatments including topiramate are thought to act partly through this mechanism.

Levetiracetam binds to the synaptic vesicle protein SV2A, decreasing calcium influx into the presynaptic terminal. It is unclear how levetiracetam suppresses seizures but it is probably related to decreased release of excitatory neurotransmitters.

The acid-base balance and maintenance of local pH is critical to normal functioning of the nervous system. Acidosis tends to increase the seizure threshold. A minor part of topiramate's mechanism of action is as a carbonic anhydrase inhibitor. Inhibition of carbonic anhydrase enzyme produces a localised acidosis by increasing concentration of hydrogen ions intracellularly. The potassium ions shift to the extracellular compartment to buffer this acidosis. This event results in hyperpolarisation and an increase in seizure threshold of the cells.

Syllabus Mapping

Neurology and neurodisability

* understand the physiological basis of brain function and how this relates to electrical activity, including that seen on the EEG
* understand the pharmacology of agents commonly used in neurological disease, including antiepileptic drugs

Pharmacology, poisoning and accidents

* understand the mode of action, physiological and metabolic mechanisms of therapeutic agents, including intravenous fluids
* understand the planned and undesired effects of therapeutic agents

References

1. Perucca E. An introduction to antiepileptic drugs. *Epilepsia* 2005;**46**:31-7.

2. Stafstro CE. Mechanisms of action of antiepileptic drugs: the search for synergy. *Curr Opin Neurol* 2010;**23**:157–163.

3. Theodore WH, Rogawski MA.(2007) Epilepsy: mechanisms of drug action and clinical treatment. In, Sibley DR, Hanin I, Kuhar M and Skolnick P, eds. *Handbook of Contemporary Neuropharmacology* , John Wiley & Sons, Hoboken, New Jersey, pp. 403–441.

4. Kwan P, Sills GJ, Brodie MJ. The mechanisms of action of commonly used antiepileptic drugs *Pharmacology & Therapeutics* 2001;**90**:21-34.

5. Sills G. (2011) Mechanisms of action of antiepileptic drugs [Online], Available: http://www. epilepsysociety.org.uk/Forprofessionals/Articles [accessed 2nd March 2013].

Chapter 43: A child on a diet for epilepsy
Dr Joia de Sa

A 7 year old boy is admitted to the children's emergency department with a 1 day history of lethargy followed by a prolonged seizure (20 minutes) at home. He has a background of complex epilepsy with several different seizure types and takes sodium valproate, levetiracetam and clobazam. His parents tell you he was started on a ketogenic diet one month ago and until this morning had been seizure free for 2 weeks. On assessment he is no longer fitting his airway is patent, his respiratory rate is 28 and his heart rate is 120 beats per minute. He is moaning and looks pale. His blood glucose is 3.1 mmol/L.

Q1.   What test should you immediately perform?

A.   Blood culture
B.   Blood ketones
C.   Full blood count
D.   Urine dipstick
E.   Valproate level

Q2.   The tests you have performed come back within the normal range. He is too lethargic to have his normal diet and you are asked to write up maintenance IV fluids. What should you prescribe?

A.   0.45% sodium chloride and 5% dextrose
B.   0.9% sodium chloride
C.   0.9% sodium chloride and 5% dextrose
D.   10% dextrose
E.   5% dextrose

Q3.   The following morning his parents want to discuss other treatment options with you. His MRI scan is normal but EEG shows widespread non-specific abnormalities. Which of the following additional treatments is most likely to be of benefit?

A.   Hemispherectomy
B.   Listening to classical music
C   St John's Wort
D.   Temporal lobe resection
E.   Vagal nerve stimulation

Answers and Rationale

Q1.   **B. Blood ketones**

Q2.   **B. 0.9% sodium chloride**

Q3.   **E. Vagal nerve stimulation**

The ketogenic diet has been described as early as 1921. This involves inducing a 'starvation state' in the body where the principle metabolic substrate for the body becomes fat, which is metabolised to produce ketone bodies. This ketogenic effect has been linked to improved seizure control in children with refractory epilepsy.

In a fasting state, amino acids cannot be used for energy by the brain and fatty acids cannot cross the blood-brain barrier. In this catabolic state, ketogenesis occurs in the liver, where fatty acids are converted to ketone bodies, which cross the blood-brain barrier. The most common formulations of the diet are a 4:1 or 3:1 fat to carbohydrate and protein ratio. These use long chain triglycerides as the main fat source.

The exact mechanism for control of seizures is unknown. There are several theories linking the by-products of ketogenesis to potential mechanisms where synaptic function is stabilised and neuronal excitability is decreased. These centre around chronic ketosis, increased availability of polyunsaturated fatty acids and decreased availability of glucose (1,2).

The ketogenic diet is indicated for those patients where seizures have failed to respond to adequate trials of antiepileptic medication, where the side-effects of anti-epileptic medication are intolerable and for certain epilepsy syndromes early in their course ie Lennox-Gastaut and Dravet syndrome (3). It is also indicated in glucose transporter 1 (GLUT 1) deficiency (where glucose transport across blood-brain barrier is impaired) and pyruvate dehydrogenase (PDH) deficiency (ketone bodies can bypass the enzyme deficiency). It is contra-indicated in patients who have fatty acid oxidation defects, organic acidurias, those with hyper or hypoglycaemic states, patients with hyperlipidaemia and those with feeding difficulties.

During the initiation of the diet, an initial acidotic state resolves within a few days. Glucose and ketones should be monitored and the child should be followed up regularly. It is a very demanding diet and parents need to be very rigorous in its administration. An ideal range for blood ketones is between 4 and 6 mmol/L (4).

Evaluation of the unwell child on a ketogenic diet must include a full clinical assessment and tests to include FBC, U&Es, LFTs, bicarbonate, blood gas analysis and blood or urinary ketones. Blood glucose levels must be checked 2 to 4 hourly especially if intake is decreased. However, in ketotic children blood sugar levels of >2.5 mmol/L are considered acceptable (4).

Excess ketogenesis may present as tachycardia, rapid panting breathing (Kussmaul respiration) and unexpected lethargy. This is defined as urine ketones >16 or blood ketones > 6 mmol/L. Treatment is to provide some carbohydrate to stop excess ketosis. Given the recent seizure in this child this should be done with considerable caution.

Therefore in our case, the most urgent test would be to check blood ketones. Urine dipstick would tell us about infection and ketosis, but not give an accurate assessment of their current level.

Where possible, given the points above, low carbohydrate clear fluids should be given if tolerated orally i.e. sugar-free squash. Standard oral rehydration solutions or indeed any fluids containing glucose may abruptly stop ketogenesis and precipitate prolonged seizures. If intravenous fluid therapy is required, use of 0.9% sodium chloride solution is recommended.

Most children with epilepsy respond to adequate treatment with anti-epileptics. However, there are a small minority of children, some with complex diagnoses, in whom it is difficult to achieve seizure freedom or even a decrease in seizure frequency. An understanding of alternative treatments is required and these children should be referred to tertiary centres with experience in these.

Neurosurgery should only be considered in children with refractory epilepsy where there is a clear epileptogenic focus (5,6). Risks and benefits must be weighed up and children undergo extensive pre-surgical evaluation with EEG, MRI, and newer techniques including functional MRI or SPECT imaging (a technique using a tracer to detect focal areas of increased blood flow during seizures). Patients must also undergo cognitive function testing to evaluate potential post-surgical deficits.

Other surgical techniques include hemispherectomy where there are malformations of cortical development such as hemimegalencephaly or porencephaly and in Rasmussen's encephalitis. However this technique is of most benefit when performed early to allow transfer of function to the contralateral hemisphere. Neither is likely to be benefit a 7 year old without a focal source.

Herbal treatments are discouraged while on anti-epileptic medication. In particular St John's Wort (Hypericum perforatum) has been shown to have inductive and inhibitory effects on various cytochrome P450 enzymes seeming to result in decreased bioavailability of anti-epileptic medication and therefore an increase in seizure frequency.

Vagal nerve stimulation may be helpful in many different types of refractory epilepsies (5,6). A small generator is implanted under the skin, usually in the left pectoral area, with a wire leading to the left vagus nerve. This is programmed to deliver a current at various intervals. The patient can also be given a magnet to use to manually activate a device at the onset of a seizure. The exact mechanism of action is not fully understood however improved outcomes have been reported in adults and children.

Listening to classical music, while relaxing, is not recognised as an adjunctive treatment for children with refractory epilepsy. Small studies have reported an effect of listening to Mozart's Sonata for two pianos in D Major, K448 (also known as Mozart K448) (7).

Syllabus Mapping

Neurology and Neurodisability

- understand the physiological and pathophysiological changes that occur in neurological disorders including epilepsy
- understand the scientific basis of non-pharmacological treatments for the management of neurological disorders and neurodisability eg ketogenic diet

Nutrition

- understand the scientific basis of nutrition
- know the principles and methods of dietary supplementation eg calories, vitamins, minerals

References

1. Bough RJ, Rho JM. Anticonvulsant mechanisms of the ketogenic diet. *Epilepsia* 2007;**48 (1)**:43-58.

2. Hartman AL, Vining EPG. Clinical aspects of the ketogenic diet. *Epilepsia* 2007;**48 (1)**:31-42.

3. Kossoff EH, Zupec-Kania BA, Amark PE, et al. Optimal clinical management of children receiving the ketogenic diet: recommendations of the International Ketogenic Diet Study Group. *Epilepsia* 2009;**50(2)**:304-17.

4. Elitze C, Fitzsimmons G, Sewell M, Chaffe H. Great Ormond Street Hospital for Children Guidelines on the Ketogenic Diet 2012.

5. Joshi SM, Singh RK, Shelhaas RA. Advanced treatment for childhood epilepsy: Beyond anti-seizure medications. *JAMA Pediatr* 2013;**167(1)**:76-83.

6 NICE guidance 2012. The diagnosis and management of the epilepsies in adults and children in primary and secondary care.

7. http://www.epilepsy.org.uk/info/treatment/mozart-effect. [accessed 25.03.13].

Chapter 44: A baby on a diet
Dr Nadya James

A 6 month baby girl is brought to see you with concerns over her weight gain and development. She was born at term weighing 3.6 Kg (50th – 75th centile) and is exclusively breastfed. Her parents are just starting to try weaning, but have found her reluctant to take solids. Her parents are healthy, unrelated and both are vegan. On examination she weighs 5.5 Kg (<0.4th centile), length 62 cm (0.4th – 2nd centile) and head circumference 42 cm (9th centile). She is pale and lethargic, with a degree of hypotonia, and has mild hepatosplenomegaly.

She has some blood tests performed:

Haemoglobin 8.0g/dL (ref 11-14g/dL)
Platelets 90 x10^9/L (ref 150-450 x10^9/L)
White cells 4.5 x10^9/L (ref 6-17 x10^9/L)
MCV 94 fl (ref 71-85 fl)
Sodium/potassium/urea/creatinine all within reference values
Calcium 2.15 (ref 2.25-2.75mmol/L)
Phosphate 1.75 mmol/L (ref 1.45-2.16mmol/L)
Albumin 30g/L (ref 30-50 g/L)

Q1. Which of the following is the most likely cause of her symptoms?

A.   Calcium deficiency
B.   Iron Deficiency
C.   Vitamin B12 deficiency
D.   Vitamin D deficiency
E.   Zinc deficiency

Q2. Which of the following would you advise for future pregnancies to prevent recurrence?

A.   Switch the infant to unmodified soy milk
B.   The mother to eat fortified margarine daily
C.   The mother to increase her intake of pulses and nuts
D.   The mother to increase her intake of dark green leafy vegetables
E.   The mother to take a vitamin D3 supplement daily

Answers and Rationale

Q1. **C. Vitamin B12 deficiency**
Q2. **B. The mother to eat fortified margarine daily**

Vegetarianism and veganism are now an established lifestyle choice for many people, and it is important that the clinician is aware of the impact it may have on maternal and infant nutrition. This is especially so in population areas where the predominant diet is vegetarian or vegan, such as parts of India.

In order to understand the infant's symptoms in the case study, we need to look at what happens to the balance of nutrients if we remove meat and fish from the diet (vegetarianism), and also milk and eggs (veganism). These dietary ingredients are important sources of macronutrients (protein and fats) but also micronutrients (vitamin D, calcium, iron, vitamin B12, zinc, omega-3 fatty acids, iodine, and vitamin B2).

Vitamin D is involved in calcium and phosphate regulation. Active vitamin D3 is found in oily fish, which is not part of a vegan diet. It can be synthesised in the skin when exposed to sunlight, and so levels may be lower in cultures where skin is to be kept covered or where high factor sun creams are used extensively. Vegans may also decide not to take vitamin D supplements as they are often made from fish oils. Likewise, most infant formulas use fish oil as their source of vitamin D. Subclinical vitamin D deficiency may be quite common, but severe cases present with defective bone mineralisation, osteopenia and rickets, and may have hypotonia or even the effects of hypocalcaemia which can include seizures. It would not however account for the anaemia and other findings in the case study.

Calcium comes primarily from dairy products, such as milk and cheese. Vegan sources include soy bean products, nuts, broccoli, seaweed and molasses. Many soy milk drinks and some fruit juices are also supplemented with calcium. In order to adequately absorb calcium from the diet, vitamin D is required. Calcium is essential in bone mineralisation, and has an extensive role as a neurotransmitter. Deficiency is linked to osteopenia and rickets. Hypocalcaemia also leads to abnormal neurotransmission, manifesting as muscles spasms and tetany, arrhythmias and seizures. Other findings include petechiae, hyper-reflexia, and (in those old enough to verbalise) paraesthesia or numbness of the extremities. At first glance the blood results seem to suggest a low serum calcium of 2.15mmol/L. However, remember that total measured calcium is influenced by serum albumin, and the calcium should be corrected using the formula: Corrected calcium (mmol/L) = measured total Ca (mmol/L) + 0.02 (40 - serum albumin [g/L]). Note: 40 = average albumin level in g/L. Following the formula using the examples in the case study: Corrected calcium = 2.15 + 0.02(40-30) = 2.35mmol/L. The adjusted calcium is thus within the given normal reference range.

Iron is found in rich quantities in meat, and is essential for haemopoesis. It is readily absorbed from meat products. Non-meat iron sources include fortified cereals, dried peas and beans, and dried fruit. However this form of iron is not so easily absorbed, and is best taken at the same time as a source of vitamin C (for example fruit juice). Iron is also present in breast milk. Breast milk has less iron than infant formulas, but it is in a form that is far better absorbed. Infants who drink a lot of standard cows' milk (i.e.

not an infant formula) are at particular risk of iron deficiency. Deficiency tends to lead to a microcytic hypochromic anaemia, often with low ferritin and sometimes with a thrombocytosis. Affected infants are pale, irritable, have poor appetite, and may have poor growth. Although iron deficiency could explain some of the symptoms in the infant in the case study, the blood results do not entirely fit with this.

Zinc is found in nuts, seeds, lentils, and fortified cereals. A good vegan diet would be expected to contain plenty of these foods. Deficiency is common in some parts of the world where it leads to poor feeding, diarrhoea, and skin breakdown. This would not account for the findings in the infant in the case study.

Vitamin B12 (cobalamin) is sourced from eggs, as well as meat and fish. Vegan sources of B12 include yeast extract spreads, vegetable and sunflower margarines, and fortified breakfast cereals. It is a factor involved in neurodevelopment and myelination, fatty acid synthesis, haemopoesis, and cell metabolism. It is absorbed in the terminal ileum in a process requiring intrinsic factor, from the gastric parietal cells. Deficiency can occur due to inadequate dietary intake, or secondary to other pathology such as pernicious anaemia or inflammatory bowel disease. Symptoms of B12 deficiency in infants include irritability, apathy, poor feeding, gastrointestinal disturbance, developmental delay or regression, hypotonia, pallor, mild hepatosplenomegaly, and sometimes skin pigment changes. Blood studies show a megaloblastic anaemia, often with a pancytopenia. Thus our infant in the case study would seem to be showing symptoms and signs consistent with vitamin B12 deficiency.

Having identified that the infant in the case study is most likely to have vitamin B12 deficiency, both the mother and infant will benefit from vitamin B12 supplementation. In some cases this may need to be given to the infant as an intramuscular injection initially, before switching to oral therapy.

A consultation with a dietician may help to identify any other areas of the mother's diet which need addressing, and to plan for how to manage future pregnancies. A multivitamin and mineral supplement throughout pregnancy and lactation should be combined with a balanced vegan diet. Advice may include that margarine and yeast extract are good sources of vitamin B12, and may be eaten daily throughout pregnancy and lactation. Unmodified soy milk would not be recommended over breast milk, although the family may wish to choose a soy-based infant formula if breast milk supply is declining now that the infant is over 6 months of age. The other three options (vitamin D3 supplements, eating pulses and nuts, and eating dark green leafy vegetables) may all be good general advice, but would not specifically protect against vitamin B12 deficiency.

Syllabus Mapping

Nutrition

* understand the scientific basis of nutrition
* understand the physiological basis of normal enteral nutrition and its variation throughout childhood
* know the constituents of a healthy diet at all ages, including the breast and formula feeding in infancy
* know the constitution of infant feeds commonly used in health and disease
* know the principles and methods of dietary supplementation, eg calories, vitamins, minerals

References

1. Guez S, *et al.* Severe vitamin B12 deficiency in an exclusively breastfed 5-month-old Italian infant born to a mother receiving multivitamin supplementation during pregnancy. *BMC Pediatrics* 2012;**12**:85.

2. McPhee AJ, *et al.* Vitamin B12 deficiency in a breast fed infant. *Arch Dis Child* 1988;**63**: 921-923.

3. Dror DK and Allen LH. Effect of vitamin B12 deficiency on neurodevelopment in infants: current knowledge and possible mechanisms. *Nutr Rev* 2008;**66(5)**:250-255.

4. Mantadakis E, *et al.* Seizures as initial manifestation of vitamin D-deficiency rickets in a 5-month-old exclusively breastfed infant. *Pediatr Neonatol* 2012;**53(6)**:384-6.

5. Chalouhi C *et al.* Neurological consequences of vitamin B12 deficiency and its treatment. *Pediatr Emerg Care* 2008;**24(8)**:538-41.

Chapter 45: A baby who can't drink milk
Dr Richard Burridge, Dr Vasanta Nanduri

A 4 month old boy had been exclusively breast fed until the age of 3 months when standard infant formula was introduced. His parents noticed that after giving the formula milk, he developed a red blotchy rash over his face and torso within a few minutes. They felt his lips became slightly swollen. He also vomited several times. There were no respiratory symptoms noted.

His mother is tearful and explains that she is unable to continue breastfeeding.

Q1. What is the most likely underlying cause of these symptoms?

A.   Frey's syndrome (auriculotemporal syndrome)

B.   IgE-mediated reaction to cow's milk protein

C.   IgE-mediated reaction to latex

D.   Lactase deficiency

E.   Mastocytosis

Q2. Which of the following would be most likely to result in an improvement of symptoms?

A.   Extensively hydrolysed infant formula

B.   Goat's milk based infant formula

C.   Lactose-free infant formula

D.   Latex-free teats

E.   Regular non-sedating antihistamine

Answers and Rationale

Q1.   B. IgE-mediated reaction to cow's milk protein
Q2.   A. Extensively hydrolysed infant formula

Whilst both are common lactose intolerance and cow's milk protein allergy are distinct entities. Lactose intolerance is caused by a partial or complete deficiency in lactase. Lactose is a disaccharide found in all mammalian milk and is normally broken down into glucose and galactose in the small intestine by lactase. Glucose and galactose are readily absorbed. Lactase deficiency results in lactose being broken down by bacteria in the large intestine leading to the production of hydrogen and methane. These gases cause abdominal distension, flatus and explosive diarrhoea.

There are three main types of lactose intolerance: Congenital absence of lactase is very rare and results in diarrhoea and faltering growth from the first exposure to lactose (usually from breast milk). This is an autosomal recessive condition and is seen in specific ethnic groups (Finland and Russia); Primary lactose intolerance which is common. It is genetic, with varying regulation of lactase enzyme gene expression. It generally presents in adult life but can occur in any age, normally over the age of 2 years, when lactase production naturally decreases in response to decreasing reliance on milk and dairy in the diet; Secondary lactose intolerance is ubiquitous and results from inflammation or structural damage of intestinal villi, leading to reduced lactase enzyme production. This commonly occurs following gastroenteritis, parasitic gut infection or any other enteropathy. It is usually transient and improves when the gut villi have been regenerated.

Diagnosis is made clinically by the elimination and re-introduction of lactose. As lactose is incompletely absorbed then stools will contain reducing sugars and hydrogen will be present in the breath following exposure to lactose. Any stool samples need to be tested within 1-2 hours as lactose continues to be broken down by gut bacteria after elimination. Provision of a lactose-free formula or substitution of mammal-based milk with a vegetable-based product (soya, oat) will alleviate symptoms.

Adverse reactions or hypersensitivities can be divided into non-immune mediated and immune mediated. Non immune mediated reactions to the constituents of milk are often referred to as intolerance, whilst immune mediated reactions are referred to as allergy. Allergic reactions may be IgE-mediated immediate onset reactions (as in our case) or non-IgE-mediated delayed onset reactions.

Reactions to cow's milk protein occur in 2-3% of young children (1). Immediate symptoms will generally occur within minutes of exposure. They range from mild symptoms such as urticaria with or without angiooedema to severe/life threatening anaphylaxis with respiratory or cardiovascular involvement (see Chapter 28). Diagnosis is made by the history of immediate onset allergic symptoms following ingestion and evidence of sensitisation via skin prick or blood specific IgE testing. Non–IgE mediated cow's milk allergy is often more difficult to diagnose as it does not cause these immediate effects and IgE-based RAST tests or skin prick testing will be negative. Diagnosis is confirmed by removal from the diet and subsequent re-exposure. Non-IgE-mediated disorders usually involve T-Cells or eosinophils. They present with gastrointestinal symptoms such as gastro-oesophageal reflux, diarrhoea, or constipation, as well as colic. Respiratory symptoms and anaphylaxis are rare. Associated atopic eczema is relatively common.

Management is strict avoidance cow's milk. In non-weaned breast fed babies, a strict maternal cow's milk-free diet may occasionally be required. The first line treatment is with a 2 – 6 week trial of an extensively hydrolysed formula (eHF) (2). A documented improvement of symptoms, ideally with evidence of worsening with re-challenge is diagnostic. This is effective in 90% of cases. Dietician input is suggested with paediatric follow up. Those who fail to respond to an eHF or have more severe symptoms can be offered a trial of an amino acid based formula. Up to 90% of affected children will lose their reactivity to milk by the age of 3 years.

Goat's milk protein is structurally very similar to cow's milk protein and more than 90% of individuals who are allergic to cow's milk will also react to goat's milk (3). Therefore goat's milk formula would be unlikely to help. Mastocytosis is a much rarer condition. There are two main forms, cutaneous and systemic. Cutaneous mastocytosis usually affects a localised area of the skin and is more common in children. Gentle pressure on the affected area leads to immediate local mast cell degranulation with swelling and urticaria. Systemic mastocytosis is quite rare in young children and does not fit the clinical features observed in our case. Frey's syndrome is a very rare condition which results in flushing and sweating of one side of the face during feeds. It is worse with foods that provoke intense salivation as it results from damage (often at birth following instrumental delivery) to the auriculotemporal branch of the trigeminal nerve. As a result of severance and inappropriate regeneration, the parasympathetic nerve fibres may switch course to the skin, resulting in flushing and sweating in the anticipation of eating, instead of the normal salivatory response.

Whilst latex is a relatively common cause of allergy in later life it is rarely seen as a trigger in early infancy. Most infant teats are in fact made of silicone, although specialist latex teats are available. A basic understanding of the constituents of infant feeds is important for paediatricians.

Protein: Whey and Casein are the main source of protein in human milk. Colostrum is mainly whey, and the ratio of whey to casein moves towards 50:50 later in lactation. First infant formulas, based on cow's milk, have their whey:casein ratio altered to around 60:40 in line with human milk early in lactation. α-lactalbumin and β-lactoglobulin are the main whey proteins in human milk. Cow's milk has less α-lactalbumin than human milk and some artificial formulas supplement this.

Carbohydrate: The main carbohydrate in both human milk and cows' milk is lactose. Lactose free or reduced lactose milks may derive their carbohydrate from maize or potatoes, or other sugars such as glucose, sucrose or corn syrups.

Fat: Fat supplies up to 50% of the energy in breast fed infants. The amount of fat in breast milk changes during the feed, and during the lactation period. Infant formulas normally contain fat from vegetable oils that supply around 50% of dietary energy.

Nucleotides: Nucleotides are synthesised from amino acids in the body to form DNA and RNA. Colostrum has a high concentration of nucleotides and this reduces over the first 4 weeks of lactation. All standard infant formulas are supplemented with nucleotides.

Long chain polyunsaturated fatty acids (LCPs): These are found in small quantities in human milk and are found in high concentrations in neural tissue and the retina. Whilst they can be synthesised in the body, many infant formulas are now supplemented with LCPs however evidence of benefit is lacking.

Vitamins and minerals: Are better absorbed from human milk than from cows' milk formulae. As a result, higher concentrations are required in infant formula than are present in human milk (4).

Alternatives to Standard Cow's Milk Based Infant Formula

Soy Milk Formula: the protein source being the soya bean. The source of carbohydrate is normally glucose, sucrose or corn syrup (lactose free). Soy milk is not recommended in male infants under 6 months of age as they contain phyto-oestrogens. Soy-based formulas are not currently recommended for treatment of CMPA as 10-15% of infants with IgE-mediated CMPA also have soy allergy. In Non-IgE mediated CMPA cross-reactions may occur in 50%.

Extensively Hydrolysed Formulas (eHF): the protein source is hydrolysed cow's milk protein. The carbohydrate source is usually corn syrup and modified corn starch (making the milk lactose and sucrose free). There is some residual β-lactoglobulin in eHF which may explain why some infants who have persistent symptoms on this preparation.

Amino Acid Formulas: the protein source is 100% amino acids. The carbohydrate source is normally corn syrup or sucrose.

Syllabus Mapping

Gastroenterology and Hepatology

- understand the physiological basis of normal gut including absorption and secretion
- know the genetic and environmental factors in the aetiology of gut disease
- understand the pharmacological basis of therapy in gut and liver disorders

Infection, Immunity and Allergy

- know the genetic and environmental factors in the aetiology of allergic disorders

Nutrition

- know the constitution of infant feeds commonly used in health and disease
- know the principles of nutritional management in childhood disease

References

1. Du Toit G, Meyer R, Shah N et al. Identifying and managing cow's milk protein allergy. *Arch Dis Child Educ Pract Ed* 2010;**95**:134-44.
2. National Institute for Health and Clinical Excellence. CG116. *Food allergy in children and young people.* London: 2011.
3. Sicherer SH. Clinical implications of cross-reactive food allergens. *J Allergy Clin Immunol* 2001;**108**:881-890.
4. Crawley H, Westland S. *Infant Milks in the UK: A Practical Guide for Health Professionals.* First Steps Nutrition Trust. November 2012.

Chapter 46: A teenager with brain stem death following trauma Dr Lynn Sinitsky

A 14 year old boy was admitted to the paediatric intensive care unit (PICU) following a road traffic collision. He was a pedestrian hit by a vehicle travelling at 50mph while crossing a road. At the scene, paramedics noted that he made no respiratory effort, his heart rate was 90 beats per minute and his Glasgow coma score (GCS) was 3. He has remained cardiovascularly stable and has required no sedation or paralysing agents. 48 hours later he continues to make no spontaneous respiratory effort and does not cough or gag with deep suctioning. His pupils are 6mm and unresponsive.

The PICU consultant explained to the boy's family that the severe damage caused by the head injury was unlikely to be compatible with life and discussed brain stem death and organ donation with the family. The parents were prepared to accept a diagnosis of brain stem death and wanted to discuss organ donation further with the local transplant team coordinator. The boy was eligible for organ donation. Brain stem death testing was conducted according to protocol. All his brain stem reflexes were absent and the boy was pronounced brain stem dead. He went on to become a heart, lung and kidney donor.

Q1. Which ONE of the following is a function of the brain stem?

A.   Coordination of motor activity
B.   Deep tendon reflexes
C.   Memory
D.   Olfaction
E.   Respiratory drive

Q2. The pupillary light reflex tests for which of the following cranial nerve(s)?

A.   Cranial nerve I
B.   Cranial nerves II and III
C.   Cranial nerves II, III, IV and VI
D.   Cranial nerve III
E.   Cranial nerves III, IV and VI

Q3. The gag reflex tests for which of the following cranial nerve(s)?

A.   Cranial nerve V
B.   Cranial nerve VII
C.   Cranial nerve VIII and IX
D.   Cranial nerve IX and X
E.   Cranial nerves X, XI and XII

Answers and Rationale

Q1.   **E. Respiratory drive**
Q2.   **B. Cranial nerves II and III**
Q3.   **D. Cranial nerves IX and X**

The 'brain death criteria' proposed by the Conference of Royal Colleges and Faculties of the United Kingdom in 1976 and 1979 have subsequently become adopted as part of the law in England and Northern Ireland courts for the diagnosis of death (1). Brain stem death is regarded as 'irreversible loss of the capacity for consciousness, combined with irreversible loss of the capacity to breathe', that is the coexistence of coma and apnoea. The irreversible cessation of brain stem function will ultimately result in the irreversible loss of the necessary functions for human existence including the cessation of the heartbeat, although the time taken for this to occur varies from hours to days or even weeks. However, for many families the concept of brain stem death is still difficult to understand. They may only accept an individual has died once the heart has stopped beating, a belief shared by some religions as well. An understanding of the process and physiology is important for paediatricians.

The brain stem extends from the upper cervical spinal cord to the diencephalon of the cerebrum. It is divided into three parts: medulla oblongata, pons and midbrain. The functions of the brain stem are: (a) conduction of information. All motor and sensory (except olfaction and vision) pathways pass through the brainstem. (b) Autonomic function including respiratory drive, heart rate, blood pressure maintenance, digestion, micturation and sleeping. These include arousal mechanisms for awareness and consciousness. (c) Origin of the nuclei for cranial nerves III-XII.

The three conditions which need to be fulfilled in order to consider a diagnosis of brain stem death are: 1. Irreversible cause of brain injury, 2. Coma and 3. Ventilator dependency as spontaneous ventilation is inadequate or absent.

There are many potential causes of irreversible brain injury. Examples include traumatic head injury, spontaneous intracranial haemorrhage, intracranial tumour, meningitis or encephalitis and cerebral hypoxia due to cardiorespiratory arrest or severe circulatory insufficiency. Drugs, hypothermia and potentially reversible circulatory, metabolic and endocrine disturbances must be excluded as potential causes for unconsciousness and/or respiratory depression. Narcotics, barbituates and opiates have a direct effect on the respiratory centre, weakening the effect of elevated carbon dioxide levels on the respiratory drive. If paralysing agents were given, reversal of neuromuscular blockade must be demonstrated by the presence of peripheral reflexes or response to nerve stimulation.

Often body temperature is low in patients with brain stem injury because central body temperature regulation is dysfunctional. Brain stem reflexes fail at core body temperatures <32°C. Therefore it is recommended that a patient is warmed if necessary to a central body temperature >35°C before brain stem tests are conducted.

Diagnosis of brain stem death
In 1998 the UK Department of Health published a code of practice for the diagnosis of brain stem death

(2). This also includes guidelines for the identification and management of potential organ and tissue donors. Discussion of organ donation is an important part of the process of diagnosing brain stem death as the decision for organ donation should be made prior to withdrawal of mechanical support.

In 1991 a report from a working party of the British Paediatric Association, supported by the Council of the Royal College of Physicians, recommended that in children over the age of 2 months, the brain stem death criteria should be the same as those in adults (3). There are different rules and legislation across the world reflecting cultural differences and a rapidly developing evidence base. In the UK, there are three conditions that need to be fulfilled before a diagnosis of brain stem death can be considered. Once all three conditions are met, the diagnosis of brain stem death is made following neurological examination of brain stem reflexes. Two sets of tests should always be performed by experienced competent and impartial observers (must have been qualified for more than five years) to remove the risk of observer error. In children the neurological examination should be carried out separately by two experienced medical practitioners of consultant or senior registrar status: one should normally be a paediatrician or have experience working with children, one should be a consultant and one not primarily involved in the child's care. No set interval between assessments is given but an interval of 12-24 hours is suggested. The concept of brain stem death in preterm infants (<37 weeks) is inappropriate. Brain stem reflexes may be immature and preclude diagnosis based upon clinical examination.

Persistent absence of all of the following brain stem reflexes is consistent with a diagnosis of brain stem death:

1. The pupils are fixed in diameter and do not respond to sharp changes in the intensity of incident light. This tests cranial nerves II and III.

2. There is no corneal reflex. There is no blinking response when touching the cornea, for example with cotton wool. This tests cranial nerves V and VII. It is important that this assessment is performed with care to avoid trauma to the cornea, one of the tissues that can be retrieved from an organ donor.

3. The vestibulo-ocular reflexes are absent. No eye movements are seen during or following the slow injection of at least 50mls of ice cold water over one minute into each external auditory meatus in turn. This tests cranial nerves III, IV, VI and VIII. Before this test can be performed, the tympanic membrane must be clearly visualised and the head should be flexed at 30°.

4. No motor responses within the cranial nerve distribution can be elicited by adequate stimulation of any somatic area. There is no limb response to supraorbital pressure. This tests cranial nerves VII, XI, XII and whether the motor pathways that pass through the brain stem are intact.

5. There is no gag reflex or reflex response to bronchial stimulation by suction catheter placed down the endotracheal tube or a tongue depressor placed in the posterior pharynx under direct vision. This tests cranial nerves IX and X.

6. No respiratory movements occur when the patient is disconnected from the mechanical ventilator

(the apnoea test). During this test it is necessary for the arterial carbon dioxide to exceed the threshold for respiratory stimulation, that is, the PaCO2 should reach 6.65kPa (50mmHg). This tests the function of the respiratory centre located in the medulla oblongata. Carbon dioxide receptors within the respiratory centre play an important role in driving respiration. Hypoxia during the disconnection should be prevented by pre-oxygenating with 100% oxygen for 10 minutes prior to disconnection and then delivering oxygen at 6L/min through a catheter in the trachea. The apnoea test should be terminated if there is hypoxia or hypotension. Patients with pre-existing chronic respiratory disease may be responsive only to supra-normal levels of carbon dioxide or depend upon a hypoxic drive. These special cases should be managed in consultation with an expert in respiratory disease.

Ancillary investigations are not required to establish a diagnosis of brain stem death.

Syllabus Mapping

This question links to the syllabus under four headings:

Neurology and Neurodisability, Ophthalmology, Palliative care and Ethics and Pharmacology, Poisoning and Accidents

- know the anatomy and understand the physiology of the central and peripheral nervous systems
- know the physiology of the eye and its movement e.g. pupillary reflexes
- understand the physiology of brainstem death
- understand the physiological and metabolic mechanisms and consequences of accidents including trauma, drowning, inhalation

References

1. Conference of Medical Royal Colleges and their Faculties in the United Kingdom. Diagnosis of brain-stem death. *Lancet* 1976;**2**:1069-70.

2. Working Group of Department of Health. A code of practice for the diagnosis of brain stem death including guidelines for the identification and management of potential organ and tissue donors. Department of Health March 1998.

3. Conference of Medical Royal Colleges and their Faculties in the United Kingdom. Diagnosis of brain stem death in infants and children. London British Paediatric Association 1991.

4. Pallis C. ABC of brain stem death. Reappraising death. *BMJ* 1982;**285**:1409-12.

Chapter 47: Mode of action of paracetamol
Dr Michelle Hills

A four week old boy born at term was admitted to the paediatric unit with projectile non-bilious, post prandial vomiting and mild dehydration. His parents and 3 year old sister have a viral illness with low grade fever, coryza and cough. The paediatrician having witnessed the projectile vomiting arranged a test feed and then an ultrasound which confirmed the diagnosis of infantile hypertrophic pyloric stenosis. A nasogastric tube was placed and intravenous fluids commenced. After discussion with the regional paediatric surgical centre it was agreed that the child would be transferred the following day to the surgical centre.

He also developed a low grade fever and mild coryzal symptoms similar to his relatives and oral paracetamol was prescribed as an antipyretic.

Q1. Why will paracetamol not be an effective antipyretic for this patient?

A.   Alkalosis
B.   Elevated cyclooxygenase levels
C.   Elevated prostaglandin H2 levels
D.   Hypochloraemia
E.   Inaccessible site of absorption

Q2. What drug should be given to this patient at this time?

A.   Aspirin
B.   Double the standard dose of oral paracetamol
C.   Ibuprofen
D.   Morphine
E.   No drug required

Q3. Paracetamol in infancy has been shown to:

A.   Be ineffective as an analgesic
B.   Be ineffective as an antipyretic
C.   Cause Reye's syndrome
D.   Lower seizure threshold
E.   Reduce the effectiveness of immunisation

Answers and Rationale

Q1.   E. Inaccessible site of absorption
Q2.   E. No drug required
Q3.   E. Reduce the effectiveness of immunisation

To comprehend the ineffectiveness of paracetamol with pyloric stenosis it is important to consider the science behind the diagnosis as well as the pharmacodynamics and pharmacokinetics of the proposed treatment. Poor understanding of the science would lead to inappropriate management of this boy.

Pyloric stenosis is a narrowing of the outlet of the stomach to the duodenum due to hypertrophy of the pylorus muscle. Stomach contents are unable to pass lower into the gastrointestinal tract. Vomiting of stomach contents (without duodenal contents) causes a loss of hydrochloric acid and potassium (K^+, H^+ and Cl^- ions) leading to a classical biochemical picture of hypokalaemic hypochloraemic alkalosis. Pyloric stenosis does not alter prostaglandin or cyclooxygenase levels. Moreover, they are not fundamentally affected by this child's age. This eliminates B. and C. as possible answers to question 1 but knowledge of paracetamol is required to determine which is the correct answer from the other options.

Despite having been used extensively and effectively for numerous years, the action of paracetamol is still not completely clear (1). Non steroidal anti inflammatory drugs (NSAIDS) and paracetamol are analgesic and antipyretic drugs. Unlike other NSAIDs, paracetamol does not have significant anti-inflammatory or anti platelet properties. NSAIDS work by inhibiting cyclooxygenase (COX) enzymes and therefore decrease the synthesis of prostaglandin H2 from arachadonic acid. Prostaglandin H2 is pivotal in the inflammatory pathway as it is converted into further prostaglandins (which modulate immune function and cause vascular dilatation) and thromboaxane (which causes platelet aggregation and platelet constriction). COX 1 is a constitutive enzyme found in most cells whereas COX 2 is the inducible form abundant in cells where there is inflammation. Paracetamol is a weak inhibitor of both COX 1 and 2 however in vivo appears to function as a selective COX 2 inhibitor (1). COX 3 (a splice variant of COX 1) has been suggested to be the site of action of paracetamol but it is unclear how clinically significant this is (1).

Although the primary site of action of paracetamol may be inhibition of prostaglandins it is believed that paracetamol works centrally through inhibition of prostaglandin synthesis in the hypothalamus, blocking spinal hyperalgesia mediated by NMDA and Substance P and due to the activation of descending serotonergic pathways (2,3).

Paracetamol is metabolised in the liver. In older children and adults approximately half is turned into a glucuronide, approximate a third into a sulphate and the rest is metabolised by the P450 cytochrome system into NAPQI (N acetyl β benzoquinone imine) which is hepatotoxic if it is not inactivated by being conjugated with glutathione (3). In neonates sulphonation is the predominant method of inactivation. In overdose, glutathione is used up. Children at risk from overdose can be identified by plasma concentration related to the time of ingestion providing at least four hours has passed (earlier results can be misleading) (4) and should be treated with acetylcysteine which acts as a glutathione replacement and scavenges free radicals, binding NAPQI directly.

Orally administered paracetamol is well absorbed from the duodenum but is not absorbed from the stomach. There is a relationship between gastric emptying and absorption. Drugs which increase gastric emptying such as metoclopramide increase absorption (5). As paracetamol is not absorbed in the stomach it is used as a marker of gastric emptying in some studies. In pyloric stenosis paracetamol is unable to reach the duodenum, the site of absorption so the drug is ineffective.

Question 2 acknowledges that paracetamol is a poor choice for this patient and asks us to consider how we would clinically manage this patient. Aspirin is absorbed in the stomach (6) so would work in pyloric stenosis however this should be avoided in children due to the increased risk of Reye's syndrome. Doubling the dose of paracetamol would not help as the drug would still not reach the site of absorption. Also, if the diagnosis was incorrect or incomplete and paracetamol did reach the site of absorption, overdose could result. Ibuprofen is not well absorbed from the stomach either usually being absorbed further down the GI tract. Morphine is a strong analgesic drug and this patient is not in pain so should not be considered.

Unless the child seemed unwell from the coryzal symptoms no medication may be required anyway (Option E). Antipyretic agents should not routinely be used with the sole aim of reducing body temperature in children with fever who are otherwise well (7).

It is postulated that fever may improve immunological responses and hinder microorganisms and it certainly has been shown to reduce the effectiveness of childhood immunisations when used routinely (8). If however the baby was distressed or unwell with an increasing temperature, paracetamol could be administered as an analgesic and antipyretic, intravenously or rectally.

Syllabus Mapping

Pharmacology, poisoning and accidents

* understand the mode of action, physiological and metabolic mechanisms of therapeutic agents, including intravenous fluids
* understand the planned and undesired effects of therapeutic agents
* understand the pharmacokinetics of commonly used medicines and the relationship to renal and other organ function

Musculoskeletal

* understand the pharmacology of agents, including monoclonal antibodies, used in the treatment of musculoskeletal disease

References

1. Graham, GG, Scott, KF. Mechanism of Action of Paracetamol. *Am J Therapeut* 2005; **12**: 46-55.

2. Bennett, PN, Morris, MJ, Sharma, P. (2012) *Clinical Pharmacology*. Edinburgh: Elsevier.

3. Drake, R. and Hain, R. (2006) Pain – pharmacological management In Goldman A., Hain, R. and Liben, S. *Oxford Textbook of Palliative Care for Children*. New York: Oxford University Press.

4. Paediatric Formulary Committee (2010). *BNF for Children.* London: BMJ Publishing Group, Pharmaceutical Press, and RCPCH Publications.

5. Ritter, JM, Lewis, LD, Mant, TGK and Ferro, A. (2008). *A Textbook of Clinical Pharmacology and Therapeutics.* London: Hodder Arnold.

6. Rang, HP, Dale, MM, Ritter, JM, Flower, RJ and Henderson, G. (2007) *Rang and Dale's Pharmacology.* Edinburgh: Elsevier.

7. National Institute for Clinical Excellence (2007) *Feverish illness in children - Assessment and initial management in children younger than 5 years (CG47),* [online] Available at: <www.nice.org.uk/guidance/CG47> [Accessed 01 February 2013]

8. Prymula R, Siegrist C-A, Chlibek R, et al. Effect of prophylactic paracetamol administration at the time of vaccination on febrile reactions and antibody responses in children: two open-label, randomised controlled trials. *Lancet* 2009;**374**:1339-135.

Chapter 48: An uncommunicative teenager who has taken an overdose Dr Mark Anderson

The following is a list of drugs and household substances:

A.   Aspirin
B.   Codeine
C.   Ethylene glycol
D.   Gamma-hydroxybutyrate
E.   Hydrogen peroxide
F.   Ibuprofen
G.   Paracetamol
H.   Warfarin

A 14 year old girl presents having deliberately ingested an unidentified substance an uncertain time ago. Select the most likely substance from the above list that would result in the following biochemical abnormalities:

Q1.   Arterial blood gas: pH 7.16   pCO2   3.1kPa   pO2 9.8kPa   HCO3   8meq/L   Base excess -18 Renal function: Sodium   139mmol/L Potassium   4.5mmol/L   Chloride   106meq/L Urea   8.2mmol/L Creatinine   88μmol/L Liver function: ALT 45U/L   ALP 120U/L   Bilirubin 17μmol/L   INR 1.2   Lactate 4mmol/L

Q2.   Arterial blood gas: pH 7.30   pCO2   4.8kPa pO2 9.8kPa HCO3   17meq/L   Base excess -8.1 Renal function: Sodium   137mmol/L Potassium   3.5mmol/L   Chloride   108meq/L   Urea   6.2mmol/L Creatinine   62μmol/L   Liver function: ALT 2546U/L ALP 347U/L Bilirubin 44μmol/L INR 3.2 Lactate 9mmol/L

Q3.   Arterial blood gas: pH 7.48   pCO2   2.9kPa   pO2 11.2kPa   HCO3   13meq/L   Base excess -10 Renal function: Sodium   138mmol/L Potassium   3.2mmol/L   Chloride   106meq/L   Urea   8.2mmol/L Creatinine   58μmol/L   Liver function: ALT 46U/L   ALP 190U/L   Bilirubin 14μmol/L   INR 1.2   Lactate 9mmol/L

Answers and Rationale

Q1. **C. Ethylene glycol**

Q2. **G. Paracetamol**

Q3. **A. Aspirin**

Deliberate ingestion of a potentially toxic substance is a relatively common reason for young people to present to paediatric services. Fortunately, the offending substance is usually known, but on occasion, the young person is unwilling, or unable, to admit to what they have ingested. In addition, toxicological diagnoses should be considered in children of all ages presenting with an unexplained depressed conscious level. There are very few specifically toxicological laboratory tests that are useful in acute poisoning, especially following delayed presentation and the standard urine screen is often not available in the time frame required to alter management. However, certain agents are associated with specific patterns of biochemical abnormalities and it is important to recognise these and understand why they occur.

Blood gas analysis is a useful test in the assessment of the potentially poisoned patient. Metabolic acidosis is a relatively common finding in more severe poisoning events; in conjunction with other basic laboratory investigations, interpreting the blood gas analysis correctly can provide strong supporting or confirmatory evidence of the offending substance in a poisoning event.

In the poisoned patient with a metabolic acidosis, calculation of the anion gap is of particular import. The anion gap provides an representation of the unmeasured ions present in plasma and is calculated as follows:

$$\text{Anion Gap} = ([Na^+] + [K^+]) - ([HCO_3^-] + [Cl^-])$$

It is sometimes calculated without the inclusion of the potassium ions, which affects the normal range. In general, a normal anion gap is considered to be 3 - 11mEq/L. As plasma is electrochemically neutral, this indicates that in normal health, there are more measureable cations than anions. An elevated anion gap indicates that, usually due to disease, there is an excess of (routinely) unmeasured anions. These anions can be endogenous (e.g. lactate, ketoacids) or exogenous (e.g. methanol, isoniazid).

This information, in the context of the clinical scenario of a young person who has ingested a potentially toxic substance, allows interpretation of the various laboratory results profiles given in the question above.

In the first scenario, the results demonstrate a metabolic acidosis with an elevated anion gap of 29.5mEq/L. The concentrations of the other measured anions provided (lactate, urea) are not especially elevated and this would indicate the presence of an unmeasured anion. Of the options provided in the list, the most likely is the toxic alcohol, ethylene glycol. A severe anion gap metabolic acidosis is classical of ethylene glycol poisoning. It develops as a result of accumulation of glycolic acid. Point of care lactate concentration can be elevated as a result of a reaction of the lactate electrode to glycolate (1).

The initial features of ethylene glycol intoxication are similar to those caused by ethanol, but progress over 4-12 hours to tachypnoea, tachycardia, hypertension and eventually shock, coma and death. Acute renal failure may also occur. The toxic effects are primarily a result of the metabolites. Ethylene glycol is metabolised by alcohol dehydrogenase and subsequently by aldehyde dehydrogenase to produce glycolic acid. This is in turn converted to glyoxylic acid and oxalic acid. Treatment of ethylene glycol intoxication is achieved by competitive inhibition of alcohol dehydrogenase by either ethanol or fomepizole. Fomepizole is to be preferred as its adverse effect profile is better than ethanol. The use of either agent prolongs the elimination half-life of ethylene glycol from approximately 3 hours to around 17 hours. Haemodialysis may be used in combination with fomepizole to good effect.

In the second scenario, the results demonstrate a metabolic acidosis with an elevated anion gap of 15.5mEq/L. However, the plasma lactate concentration is also elevated at 9mmol/L which would account for this. The remainder of the results exhibit a significant hepatic dysfunction and therefore the most likely culprit from the list provided is paracetamol. Lactic acidosis is not unusual in significant paracetamol poisoning and can occur as an early phenomenon in the case of massive paracetamol ingestion or later (as in this scenario) as a result of hepatic dysfunction (2).

Approximately 90% of the therapeutic paracetamol dose undergoes hepatic glucuronidation or sulfation. The remainder is metabolised by the cytochrome P450 oxidase system to produce the potentially toxic metabolite N-acetylbenzoquinoneimine (NAPQI). Under normal circumstances, this is bound by intracellular glutathione and detoxified to form cysteine and mercapturic acid conjugates. However, in the case of overdose, the glucuronidation and sulfation pathways become saturated and the intracellular glutathione is rapidly depleted leading to a rise in the intracellular concentrations of NAPQI which causes widespread hepatocyte damage. N-acetylcysteine (NAC), the treatment for paracetamol overdose, ameliorates NAPQI toxicity by a number of proposed mechanisms, including direct binding of NAPQI and reduction back to paracetamol, provision of inorganic sulphate for glutathione synthesis and increasing glutathione availability. For maximum beneficial effect it should be administered within 8 hours of an acute paracetamol overdose.

In the third scenario, the results demonstrate a mixed respiratory alkalosis and metabolic acidosis with an elevated anion gap of 22.2mEq/L which is partly accounted for by the elevated lactate concentration. This is a classical pattern of derangement seen in salicylate toxicity in adults and adolescents. Younger children typically present with an isolated metabolic acidosis.

Salicylates initially directly stimulate the respiratory centre of the central nervous system causing hyperventilation resulting in a respiratory alkalosis. Salicylates also uncouple oxidative phosphorylation leading to lactic acid accumulation. The resultant reduction in ATP production via this route leads to promotion of fatty acid oxidation, leading to generation of ketone bodies. The accumulation of ketone bodies and lactate lead to a metabolic acidosis later in the clinical course.

The treatment of toxicity due to salicylates is to enhance their elimination. They are effectively removed by haemodialysis. Urinary alkalinisation is also effective and is used in any symptomatic patient to reduce symptoms and prevent progression and avoid the need for haemodialysis. Salicylates exist as weak acids and, as a result, the degree of ionisation is greater at higher pHs. They are renally excreted and thus, by increasing the alkalinity of the urine in the renal tubular lumen, increased ionisation favours excretion over passive diffusion back into the blood. A 10 to 20 fold increase in renal salicylate clearance is associated with an increase in urinary pH from 5 to 8. It would appear that enhanced clearance is much more dependent upon urine pH rather than urine flow and as a result, a forced diuresis is not required (3).

Syllabus Mapping

Q1. Pharmacology, poisoning and accidents

- understand the mode of action, physiological and metabolic mechanisms and consequences of substances taken without medical advice for recreational use or self-poisoning

References

1. Pernet P, Bénéteau-Burnat B, Vaubourdolle M, Maury E, Offenstadt G. False elevation of blood lactate reveals ethylene glycol poisoning. *Am J Emerg Med* 2009;**27**:132.e1-2.

2. Shah AD, Wood DM, Dargan PI. Understanding lactic acidosis in paracetamol(acetaminophen) poisoning. *Br J Clin Pharmacol* 2011;**71**:20–28.

3. Prescott L *et al.* Diuresis or urinary alkalinisation for salicylate poisoning. *BMJ* 1982;**285**:1383-6.

Chapter 49: Who signs for Sarah? Parental responsibility in the UK Dr Lucy Shonfeld

Sarah is 15 years old. She attends the surgical day case ward for a tonsillectomy. She is accompanied by her grandmother, whom she is currently staying with as her mother often travels abroad with work. Her parents are separated, and she does not have contact with her father. Sarah appears to understand the information given to her about the procedure and is keen to proceed.

Q1. Who should consent for Sarah to have her procedure? Give the one best answer

A.   Her grandmother as she is currently her guardian
B.   No one, as her parents are not present
C.   Sarah
D.   Sarah's mother
E.   Social Care

Harry is 2 months old and has been admitted to the paediatric ward overnight following some concerns due to crying and unexplained bruising. Social Care have been involved and a formal child protection medical has been performed. He has been admitted to the ward overnight as a place of safety and is awaiting a skeletal survey

Q2. Harry's mother wishes to stay overnight with Harry. What is the best correct response?

A.   No, not under any circumstances, as there are child protection concerns
B.   Overnight stays are not allowed unless a court order is obtained by the mother
C.   She should only be allowed on the ward during the day
D.   Yes, she can stay – she retains parental responsibility for Harry
E.   Yes, but only if continuously supervised by social care

The next day a skeletal survey is performed and reveals old rib fractures, along with a fractured left humerus. A further interview with the parents reveals concerns about an inflicted injury by his parents. A care order is obtained, and following his course of treatment, Harry is discharged to foster care. Harry's mother is concerned about her rights to see him.

Q3. Which of the following is NOT true? Choose one answer.

A.   Harry's mother can expect legal advice and support
B.   Harry's mother will not be able to visit Harry due to child protection concerns
C.   Harry's mother will retain parental responsibility
D.   The Local Authority must apply to the court if it wants to end or restrict contact and prove that this is in the child's best interests
E.   The Local Authority will gain parental responsibility

Answers and Rationale

Q1. **C. Sarah**
Q2. **D. Yes, she can stay – she retains parental responsibility for Harry**
Q3. **B. Harry's mother will not be able to visit Harry due to child protection concerns**

An understanding of the law and how this relates to consent and parental responsibility is important for all paediatricians.

Consent to treatment for children

Consent to medical treatment can be made by the young person if they are assessed to be competent to do so, or if not competent consent may be made by a parent or legal guardian, or by the courts. Although a person may not be competent to consent, it is still good medical practice to involve a young person in the decision surrounding their treatment.

In order for a young person to be competent to consent to treatment, they must be capable of understanding the information given to them, to be able to weigh up the risks against the intended benefits, and to be able to come to a balanced decision.

The name given to the legal precedent which established the ability of a young person to consent to treatment in England and Wales is Fraser competence (although it is sometimes referred to as Gillick competence). This was named after a legal case which looked specifically at whether doctors should be able to give contraceptive advice or treatment to under 16-year-olds without parental consent. But since then, this principle has been more widely applied to help assess whether a child has the maturity to make their own decisions and to understand the implications of those decisions. The name Gillick derives from Mrs Victoria Gillick, who took her Local Health Authority to court in an attempt to stop girls under the age of 16 years receiving contraceptive advice or treatment without parental knowledge. The case was originally dismissed but the Court of Appeal reversed the decision. The case then went to the House of Lords, and the Law Lords (including Lord Fraser) ruled in favour of the original decision.

In the case above the young person seems to understand the procedure and therefore can be assumed to be competent to consent. Therefore consent can be given by Sarah. If Sarah was deemed not to be competent her mother, as her legal guardian, could consent to the treatment. Sarah's grandmother does not have parental capacity, therefore cannot consent for treatment.

It is good practice for the young person to discuss any proposed treatment with their parents but if they do not wish to do so, in a competent patient treatment may still go ahead.

If a child refuses any treatment it is important to carefully consider if the treatment is in their best interests. This may involve discussion with a colleague, a specialist, or defence organisation. If treatment is deemed to be in the best interests of the child and there is time to spare, ie it is not immediate life-saving treatment, then a court order may be obtained.

In an emergency life saving treatment can be given if it would be deemed in the child's best interests by a panel of experts.

Child protection and the Rights of the Parents

In a case involving child protection it is always important to continue to act in the best interests of the child and to act in a non-judgemental manner. This means that it is often in the best interests of the child to retain contact with their parents unless it is specifically felt to be detrimental to the child.

In the first part of our second case, it is unlikely from the details given that there are sufficient concerns to prevent the mother from remaining with the child. However it would be good practice for the child to be nursed close to the nursing station and any concerns made by the team looking after the child to be recorded. It is also important to be guided by the child's social worker.

When there are concerns about the child's safety, the local authority can apply to the courts for an Emergency Protection or Care Order, if it is felt that there is immediate risk of harm.

An Emergency Protection Order allows the local authority to remove the child from where he or she is living to a place of safety. The Order usually lasts for up to 8 days but it can be extended for up to 7 days. In most cases an Emergency Protection Order will be followed by care proceedings.

A Care Order gives the local authority parental responsibility for the child. The local authority can then make decisions which are necessary to safeguard and promote the child's welfare. The order does not remove parental responsibility from the parents.

If the court makes a Care Order it must also consider contact for the child with their family. The court can then decide if the parents or other relatives can have ongoing contact with a child in care. Except in emergencies, the local authority must apply to the court if it wants to end or restrict contact and prove that this is in the child's best interests. If a parent, a relative, or the child wants more contact than the local authority will allow, he or she can apply to the court.

For question 3, although parts C and E might appear at first glance to be contradictions they are in fact both correct. Whilst the local authority gains parental responsibility it is also retained by the mother. Part D is also correct; and for this reason legal advice may be required by families. In some cases a barrister is made available for each parent and the child.

Except where immediate action is required in order to protect a child, the local authority tries to work with the family in order to bring about change before starting court proceedings. This will usually involve a full assessment, provision of services and a child protection plan. The local authority will tell the parents if it is considering care proceedings. In these circumstances the parents are advised to contact a family law solicitor who is a specialist child care lawyer as soon as possible. Parents and their legal advisers can meet with social workers to discuss the best arrangements for the child. Currently legal representation is available under the legal aid scheme without charge for parents.

Syllabus Mapping

Editorial note:

Currently this question does not map to the Theory and Science Syllabus. However, this is an oversight and will be rectified in future iterations.

From 2014 onwards it will probably read something like this:

Safeguarding

- be familiar with child protection legislation in the UK
- know the current legal framework concerning consent and children for the UK
- understand the principles of child advocacy

References

1. NSPCC Factsheet: Gillick competency and Fraser guidelines http://www.nspcc.org.uk/inform/research/questions/gillick_wda61289.html

2. 0-18 Years, Guidance for all Doctors. General Medical Council. 2012

3. Judiciary of England and Wales. Guide to the Family Justice System http://www.judiciary.gov.uk/about-the-judiciary/advisory-bodies/fjc/family-justice-system/issues/Child-protection

Chapter 50: Trial design
Dr Mark Anderson

A double-blind, randomised controlled trial of a new maintenance therapy for asthma in teenagers is planned.

Q1. Which ONE of the following statements concerning trial design is correct?

A.   A crossover trial design would obviate the need for a washout period

B.   A non-inferiority trial design is required when it is ethical to use placebo

C.   A smaller expected treatment effect will result in a larger sample size

D.   Having multiple outcome measures will result in a reduced chance of detecting a spurious treatment effect

E.   Self-reported asthma control is an objective outcome measure

The trial shows a statistically significant difference (p=0.0023) between treatment and placebo for its primary outcome measure. However, analysis of baseline characteristics for the each of the trial arms reveals more young people with a lower forced expiratory volume in one second (FEV_1) in the placebo group than the treatment group and there are concerns that this may have contributed to the observed difference.

Q2. Which ONE of the following statements is most correct?

A.   All young people in both arms with an FEV_1 less than 50% of expected should be excluded from the analysis

B.   Baseline FEV_1 may be a confounder and should be corrected for in the statistical analysis

C.   The baseline characteristics should all be compared using p-values to determine whether the difference is significant; if there is a statistically significant difference it indicates that the randomisation process has failed

D.   The trial results are invalid as randomization should result in identical baseline characteristics in each trial arm

E.   The difference can be ignored because children were randomised to either active treatment or placebo

Answers and Rationale

Q1.   C. A smaller expected treatment effect will result in a larger sample size

Q2.   B. Baseline FEV1 may be a confounder and should be corrected for

The Randomised Controlled Trial (RCT) is the gold standard for clinical trials and is used to compare the effect of an intervention on a predetermined outcome measure, within a particular population of subjects. An adequate understanding of the design, analysis and conduct of clinical trials is vital to allow the paediatrician to reliably form opinions of the validity of published trial data. A well constructed RCT should provide sufficient evidence to warrant a change in clinical practice.

In an RCT, subjects must be randomly allocated to one or more intervention groups and there must be a control (comparator). The primary aim is to determine the effect of the intervention(s) in relation to the control, and in relation to each other in the case of multiple interventions. RCTs can look for: superiority – one intervention is more effective than another; equivalence – one intervention is as effective as another; or non-inferiority – one intervention is not less effective. Equivalence and non-inferiority trials are usually conducted when a new intervention has fewer adverse effects or is less expensive than existing treatments. Non-inferiority and equivalence trials typically require a smaller sample size than active comparator superiority trials; however this is not always the case as sample sizes of non-inferiority trials are very sensitive to assumptions relating to the effect of the intervention in relation to its control. The sample size can be considerably larger if the two treatments are assumed to be equivalent than if the new treatment is assumed to be slightly more effective than the active control. Non-inferiority trials may be necessary when a placebo group can not be ethically included, but the results of such trials are usually not as credible as those from a superiority trial (1).

The study arms of most trials are parallel groups i.e. each group of subjects undergoes only one intervention. Occasionally, a crossover design is used ie a single group undergoes both interventions in a random order. In crossover studies each participant acts as their own control group thus fewer participants are required. Crossover trials are appropriate for a relatively restricted set of circumstances. They may be useful for studying outcomes relating to relief of symptoms rather than cure but they are not useful where an intervention is aimed at cure or when interventions have long lasting effects. There should be no residual effect from the first intervention by the time the second intervention is received, necessitating a "washout period" to allow the effects of the first intervention to wear off.

Determining the most appropriate outcome measure for a clinical trial requires careful thought. The primary outcome measure should be well defined and appropriate to the condition under study, so that if the trial returns a positive outcome, health professionals are persuaded to change practice. Endpoints can be subjective or objective, and real or surrogate. In the asthma trial above, the following outcomes might be used as evidence of positive effect on asthma control:

* Improvement in self-reported asthma symptoms (subjective, real)
* Reduction in admissions with asthma exacerbation (objective, real)
* Improvement in lung function tests (objective, surrogate)

Outcome measures may also be single or composite. Composite outcome measures are particularly common in clinical trials of cardiovascular drugs, combining separate outcome measures (e.g. death, non-fatal stroke and non-fatal myocardial infarction), making it easier to detect a treatment effect. However, there are limitations: composite endpoints may mask evidence that an intervention has a positive effect on some, but not all, of the constituent elements of the composite; and conversely, differences in composite endpoint may result from the effect of an intervention on only one of the constituents.

Most trials define a single primary outcome measure (endpoint), with a number of secondary outcome measures. Having multiple outcome measures may seem sensible as there often a range of possible endpoints in most clinical trials. However, multiple endpoints risks confusion, as an intervention may appear to be beneficial for some outcome measures and not others. In addition, multiple outcomes increase the risk of detecting a spurious treatment effect.

The primary outcome measure is used to estimate a sample size for the study. The information required to perform this estimation is: the expected effect in the intervention group and the comparison group; the significance level (usually 5%) and the power (usually 80% or 90%). The sample size estimate will go up if the expected treatment effect gets smaller (it is more difficult to detect small differences) or if the significance level decreases or the power goes up as this will increase the possibility of detecting a treatment effect if there truly is one. The type of outcome measure also determines the most appropriate statistical test to compare the groups.

Randomisation is one of the key design elements of RCTs. Randomisation minimises confounding by ensuring the characteristics of the trial groups are similar. It also reduces bias by ensuring that trial staff are unable to predict which trial group individuals will be allocated to. In essence, randomisation should ensure that the only systematic difference between the trial groups is the intervention, and thus, any difference observed in the outcome measures is attributable to the intervention. It does not ensure identical groups.

There are a number of different methods of randomisation. Simple randomisation is analogous to a coin toss for each participant – if heads, give one intervention; if tails, give the other, although this particular method is not to be advised - using a random number list is preferable. For large trials, simple randomisation should result in similarly sized groups. In smaller trials, however, it is possible to get rather unequally sized groups by chance. This can be avoided by using block randomisation – trial participants are randomised by blocks so that, for example, for every four participants, two are allocated to each trial arm. Using simple randomisation for small trials can also result in an imbalance in the baseline characteristics of each group, some of which may have an effect on the outcome measure and therefore affect the trial results. These imbalances can be avoided during recruitment by using stratified randomisation or minimisation. Stratified randomisation involves using simple randomisation for each factor that might influence the trial outcome measure e.g. for the asthma trial, the young people might be divided into two groups based on an FEV_1 of above or below 50% and each group then randomised to each of the treatment arms. Minimisation is a method of randomisation which seeks to ensure balance between trial arms by examining the existing imbalance between the groups at the time the participant is randomised. Thus, in the asthma trial above, if after twenty participants have been randomised it is apparent that there are more participants with a low FEV$_1$ in trial arm A than B, the next participant with a low FEV$_1$ will be allocated to trial arm B and so on, until the arms are balanced. Minimisation is not truly random, as allocation can be predicted. (2)

Trial reports should contain a table showing a comparison of baseline characteristics between the trial arms. The purpose is to demonstrate that randomisation has been successful in producing similar groups, thus indicating that any differences in outcome measures are due to the interventions. On occasion, the comparison is presented with p-values for each characteristic. This is inappropriate (3). P-values examine whether the characteristics came from different distributions, whereas this is already known as the participants were randomised from the same population defined by the eligibility criteria of the trial. In large trials, seemingly statistically significant differences in baseline characteristics can emerge. They do not indicate a failure of randomisation. What is important is whether the differences are likely to alter the trial outcome measures. Ideally, differences in baseline characteristics that may distort the comparison should not occur as a result of good trial design and the use of stratification or minimisation during recruitment. However, the correct application of statistical methods, e.g. multivariate regression, can take account of potential confounders.

Syllabus Mapping

The Science of Practice

* understand the principles and use of statistical testing
* understand the principles of research methodologies

References

1. Snapinn SM. Noninferiority trials. *Curr Control Trials Cardiovasc Med* 2000;**1**:19-21

2. The CONSORT Group. Box 2 – Randomisation and minimisation. www.consort-statement.org. Accessed 1 May 2013.

3. Senn SJ. Testing for baseline balance in clinical trials. *Stat Med* 1994;**13**:1715-26.

Further Reading

Swinscow TDV (Revised by Campbell MJ) Statistics at Square One. 9th Ed. BMJ Publishing Group. Available free at http://www.bmj.com/about-bmj/resources-readers/publications/statistics-square-one

Postscript

For anyone who has completed the book. Well done. For those who have turned to the back in the hope of some more wisdom or respite then here it is.

The questions in this book range from fairly simple to excrutiatingly difficult. Candidates often leave the MRCPCH Theory and Science examination convinced that they have failed. This is because they can recall all the questions that they could not answer and several which they have simply guessed. They sometimes rail against both the exam and examiners for asking what can appear to be trivial questions.

However, there has yet to be a candidate in all of history who has scored 100% (or even close to 100%) in the written papers. Indeed, our expectation as examiners is that even the best candidates will not be able to answer all the questions. The pass mark for each exam is dependent upon the difficulty of the questions included. This is set only when each question has undergone a thorough review in terms of performance and quality. Do not worry if you did not know all the answers. Likewise, do not panic if you cannot answer all of the questions in the exam itself. This does not mean you will fail and most importantly it does not make you a bad doctor. Nonetheless, a more complete scientific knowledge will make you a better doctor.

We hope that this book will serve, in part, to illuminate candidates about how a question is generated. The discussion of each case shows how a thorough understanding of the science can improve your clinical practice and allow you as a young doctor to 'troubleshoot' when a clinical problem arises. We also hope it will inspire many of you to fall in love again with the basic science which should underpin all our practice. A thorough and more comprehensive understanding of the science we hope will translate itself into better care for children and their families.

9 781906 579098